His History, Her Story

His History, Her Story

A Survival Guide for Spouses of
Male Survivors of Sexual Abuse and Trauma

DEBRA WARNER, PSY.D.

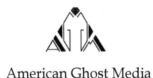

American Ghost Media

His History, Her Story, 2nd Edition

American Ghost Media, LLC
1305 Pico Blvd
Santa Monica, CA 90405

ISBN 978-0-9831635-6-5

Printed in the United States
1st Printing 2017

ATTENTION: ORGANIZATIONS & CORPORATIONS
Bulk quantity discounts for reselling, gifts or fundraising are available. For more information, please contact American Ghost Media Sales:
Sales@AmericanGhostMedia.com

Cover Design: Dave Warner

Testimonials

His History, Her Story is a must-read for intimate partners of men who suffered sexual abuse as children. A leading forensic psychologist, Dr. Debra Warner explores the topic with clinical depth while also offering practical guidance on navigating relationships from her experience as a survivor's wife. The result is a groundbreaking, comprehensive work.

Christina Hoag
co-author of *Peace in the Hood: Working with Gang Members to End the Violence*

***

A timely, indispensable treatise for the spouse, friend or supporter of an adult survivor of child abuse! Should be on every therapist's booklist, too!

Bill Murray
NAASCA.org - National Association of Adult Survivors of Child Abuse

Dedication

To the two people who are my everything: Sonya and Lawrence.

So you can know and understand our love when we are gone.

Contents

Acknowledgements

Countless times I have read book acknowledgements and wondered what people are thinking as they write the thank yous to those who have contributed to the book. I have thought, how do they choose who to thank? I have thought, how do they find the words? I have been avoiding this page, leaving it for last. Not out of fear, but out of the emotion that it is taking to write. I want to say all of those warm fuzzy sentiments, but I can't. As I write this, I am filled with sadness, thankfulness, and clarity at the same time.

First, sadness. I am filled with sadness because here I am writing this book and likely going to benefit in some way from someone else's pain. I know that I may not get rich or famous, but there will be some professional kudos that come from being a published author. I will receive admiration from someone else that has been traumatized and abused. I was not the one who struggled, but the one that experienced the secondhand effects of the struggle, and now I am writing the book. It makes me sad to know that as a woman it is likely easier for the reader to hear my journey and story than if this was coming from a man. It breaks my heart that in our society men still cannot show that type of vulnerability.

However, that sadness is what also makes me thankful. As I sat with a client recently and listened to his story, I realized I was being told the story not only because I was assigned the case, but because I am the vessel intended to be doing this work. I was thankful. I was thankful that in this world, telling me his story was likely easier because I was a woman. I was thankful because I was chosen to hear the story. I was thankful that the experience of knowing my clients, my survivors, my champions makes me a better psychologist and by far a better person.

I am also thankful that as I go home, I get to grow even more with a man who lets me be me. Every day I am surrounded by men. Every day I am giving all my emotion to other men to help them heal and every day as I walk through the door I get a kiss and a "How was your day?" I never get a jealous inquiry. One day I asked my husband why he never seems bothered by my choice of professional career and his response shocked me. He said "You have to be you. You love what you do. You understand the pain. You understand the journey men face. You saved me. They have no one else. Just be you." He then asked me, "Do you know why these guys talk to you so much?" and I said no with a dumbfounded look on my face. He said, "It is because you are so not from their world. You are 'The Brady Bunch.' You represent the world they wanted to live in and they did not get to. Yet, there you are, right there no matter what, embracing them and all their past, listening and never judging." As he said this, I realized what a blessing I have as a husband. What a strong man he is. What an honor it is to be married to a man who understands me, and has the strength to share what he has found in a wife with my chosen professional career.

So in this sadness and thankfulness I have found clarity. I know no one else has the right to tell a survivor's story but the survivors themselves. I understand now what my role is in life. I understand why I work in prisons. I understand why I work with cases no one wants. I understand I can tell the stories of survival they cannot. I understand I am the voice for the voiceless. I understand why I married the man I did. I thank God for the blessing he has given me by putting me in the position to know all the survivors that have been in my path, for making me who I am and continue to be. Therefore, this acknowledgement is for all those male survivors that have touched my heart and very soul. May I still continue to be your voice, and above all thank you for telling me your story.

Special Acknowledgements

To J. Roxann Wright: Without you this book would not have begun. Thank you for your ear and support. You are a talent.

To David Pisarra, Michael Oropollo, and American Ghost Media: Thank you for making this book happen. David Pisarra, this is why you are a Fabulous 6. Thank you for supporting and pushing me out of my comfort zone. Michael Oropollo, THANK YOU, THANK YOU, THANK YOU. You have my voice and our bond is always.

Introduction

As a former law enforcement officer who specialized in the horrendous crime of child sexual abuse, I have more than a passing knowledge of the dynamics and long-term effects on the victims. My personal experience as a survivor of sexual abuse gives me an intimate understanding of the lifetime traumas that continue to be lived by the innocent.

The direct physical effects of abuse often disappear within weeks, but the emotional, psychological, and indirect physical harms often last for decades, echoing throughout a person's life. I know that the pain, the self-loathing, the profound inability to create lasting intimacy that I faced were all results of the abuse I experienced at the hands of a man I looked up to as a mentor. When he took advantage of the situation and abused me, it set in motion relationship problems that took years of therapy and hard work to overcome.

My ultimate healing came about through the most unforeseeable of circumstances. After decades of living in fear that I would run into my mentor/abuser, I finally did. I was a prosecutor at the time and reached out to the FBI, which started an investigation that resulted in the conviction of that man and the closure of many painful chapters in my life.

I was lucky to be working in a field where therapists and experts were available for me to address my questions. The resources at my disposal were state of the art, yet they were still meager. That is why I am so happy to see that Dr. Debra Warner and her husband Dr. Robert Carey have found the courage, the dedication and the fearlessness to share their story in this book. Male survivors of child abuse, in any form, are usually told to "suck it up" or "walk it off" or, worst of all, "you got lucky." That minimization and invalidation of the trauma only serves to reinforce the trauma, and sets the stage for greater harm to that young man in the future.

When a male survivor learns that his feelings are invalidated, he'll stop expressing them. That's what I did. When a person is told that the reality they are living is not real, they will question their own abilities to judge rightly. That happened to me, and resulted in low self-esteem and self-destructive behaviors. All of this was set up by the abuser's grooming process to take advantage of the youth in the first place.

This book will help both survivors and their spouses understand and confront the myriad issues that a survivor must navigate to establish and maintain a loving relationship with themselves and with a partner. . Spouses are often confused and begin to doubt their own sanity before the full picture of abuse comes into focus. Survivors often lack both the emotional vocabulary necessary to explain the pain they feel and the tools they need to build a healthy relationship.

There is an enormous demand for this book, and I am excited to know that there is now this resource for both survivors and their spouses to begin the healing process and hopefully keep their relationship intact.

I hope that this book helps you and your spouse recover and rebuild the life that was rightfully due both of you; the life that was stolen years ago by an abuser. I know it can be done because I did it, and you can as well with the help of concerned and capable mental health professionals and resources like this book.

God bless,

James Clemente, Esq.

FBI Supervisory Special Agent (Ret.)

Foreword

Observing Her Journey

Writing a book is a complicated and lengthy endeavor. The author often goes through a deep emotional process until they cross the finish line. The final product is an amalgamation of rewrites and edits that only those who are inside the process get to witness. It is rare for an outsider to be part of this deeply internal process. But as a graduate student, I witnessed Dr. Debra Warner's journey with this book as she mentored me through my academic program. I write this foreword to let people know that this book is a true statement of someone who not only believes in her words, but actively practices them. She tells her story through the lens of love, describing her tireless efforts to champion the removal of stigma from male survivors of abuse as a testament of love for her husband.

When Dr. Warner started on this journey, she told me her goal was to write a book that would elucidate the issues that accompany marriage to a male survivor of abuse. Finding the writer's voice is difficult, and it took Dr. Warner a while to find hers. The words didn't come easily at first. She had so many things that she wanted to say, and so much passion and information for the subject that she wanted to give.

I could also see that talking about these issues from a personal perspective was harder for her than talking about them from a clinical perspective. She always wanted the love to shine through. She accomplished that by making her emotional journey with her husband the core of each topic in the book. Slowly, she found her voice with the help and guidance of a team of contributors and supportive friends and family. Her writing took form, and the book was on its way. Writing the book was also an emotional journey for her. She increased her vulnerability in talking publicly about her own experiences and her personal growth as a partner rather than as an expert clinician. Her self-awareness truly blossomed as a consequence.

This book is a testament to Dr. Warner's diligence towards the challenging goal she has set herself: removing the stigma and invisibility of the suffering of male survivors. By creating a book that is both an ally and an aide, she has provided a work for those who need help and guidance when engaging in relationships with those who have suffered. This book is an important step to bring light to this dark and taboo subject.

J. Roxann Wright, M.S.

Chapter 1

Her Story

As a psychologist working extensively in the field of male trauma and male survivors, the question I am most often asked is "Why are you so interested in male survivors and men's issues?" The short answer is that I am a male brain trapped in a pink dress. As part of my daily job, I am paid to go into prisons and other institutions and analyze the most critical, most difficult cases. I am the person who is called to solve the toughest riddles and provide treatment to the untreatable. Often I can spot the issues these men have dealt with long before they tell me.

Usually I only have one chance to get it right. It may sound strange, but once a man discloses his history of abuse to me, my goal is to get him to cry at some point in treatment. I may be the only person he has ever told this secret to, and this may be the first and last time this secret ever passes his lips. It is imperative that I provide a safe space for him to express this secret, and if he cries, I know I have succeeded. When all of those emotions that have been dammed up behind walls and mirrors begin to flood out of him, his recovery process begins.

I can always tell when a man has never disclosed his trauma to anyone, and in the case of an initial disclosure, it's important to not interrupt his flow and just listen. My process of receiving a disclosure, which has worked hundreds of times with cases all over the spectrum of severity, can be broken down into: Believe, Be Present, Acknowledge. I believe them by giving them my undivided attention. I have a ritual to help me because listening is not an innate skill of mine. I love to talk so I carry gum, nuts, or soda with me into sessions to keep my mouth occupied. As soon as they start talking, I cross my legs and become still. I do not want to distract from the flow of the disclosure. While they are in the process of disclosing to me, I am completely present with them. They have my absolute, undivided attention. I keep myself completely available and remain captive until they stop talking. Finally, I acknowledge what they have shared with me. I will say something like, "that had to be really hard for you," or I try to educate them by saying something like, "that must have been difficult for you to share; society doesn't allow men to have feelings like that." This might be the only thing I say during the entire encounter. I never try to push them along or draw out information. I mostly remain silent; they know I am waiting.

I never, under any circumstance, say, "I know how you feel." First, I don't know how they feel. I am not a man, and I have not experienced the world through their lens. A statement like that is a dismissive one and could potentially cause further trauma if they feel like I've dismissed their story or cast pity on them.

Finally, after hearing an initial disclosure, I always thank the man for telling me. If you are the person they have chosen to disclose this secret to for the first time, it is a gift. Their honesty and voluntary vulnerability is to be honored and acknowledged.

One case of an initial disclosure stands out among the many I have heard over the years. He was a young student at a nearby university. He bought a house and was working on it with the intention of flipping it for a profit. The next-door neighbor and he had been butting heads ever since the young man bought the house, for reasons that weren't exactly clear. Eventually, this escalated into a verbal altercation. The neighbor accused him of trespassing on the property. The police had a documented history of disputes between the two neighbors, and had been called to the scene several times over the last few months. Knowing this history, the young man called the police in an effort to pre-empt any further escalation. The police showed up, but because of the young man's mental health and substance abuse record, decided that he was the aggressor and began interrogating him, which led to a fight between him and the officers.

What was thought to be a good idea of calling the police before the situation escalated turned into the young man being charged with assaulting an officer. He was sentenced to two years in prison. As fate would have it, this was the same prison in which I was evaluating the psychiatric conditions of the male prisoners.

I was sitting in my office when his case came across my desk. I have worked in a number of prisons, and the psychiatric offices are generic. There are three walls of solid concrete with one wall made of glass which allows the guards to see into the room. There are two blue Rubber Maid chairs in the middle of the room with my chair positioned near the door. There is a desk with a radio on it that serves as a buzzer; if the radio is knocked over, the alarm sounds and guards rush in.

I can't work in this depressing and dehumanizing environment so I brought in pink leopard print pillows and Hello Kitty accessories – staplers, prints for the wall, stickers, door sign, pens – everything was bright pink. I brought in board games and stacked them in a corner.

The faces of the prisoners when they entered my office were priceless; it was like they were walking into another dimension. They were used to seeing nothing but institutional grey concrete walls, sometimes for years or decades. The guys told me my office had a comfort to it. It made me a real person – not a generic, sterile psychologist. It made them feel as if they were human, as well. It brought an element of personality and humanity into the environment that they rarely received elsewhere in prison.

The young man came into my office and when the initial shock at the décor wore off, he sat across from me and began telling his story. I could tell something wasn't right, but I knew he wasn't lying. I knew by the soft, indirect way in which he spoke to me and the heaviness of his eyes, which burdened us both, that there was deep pain there.

My intuition told me to ask. "Have you ever been physically or sexually abused?" I received the answer in a deafening absence of sound.

"OK, so what happened?"

"Nothing happened."

"Something obviously bothers you." I put my pen down softly on the table to show him that he had my full attention. "So, what is it?"

He got quiet, looked down, and started shaking. I knew the response he gave me next would shape him for the rest of his life, but I couldn't push him to the answer. I just remained present with him - silent. He had my attention; my silence told him that I was available for him, waiting for whatever he was going to say next. We sat like that for a while, our quiet presence filling the room. I could see a sense of urgency come over the young man, and then he came out with it: "I have a neighbor who used to pay me in drugs to do stuff with him." I paused, waiting to see if he was finished. When I knew he was done, I said, "Whether it was for drugs or not, or if you did or didn't do it, it doesn't matter. He was an adult and you were a child, and that is messed up."

He backtracked quickly. "But nothing ever happened!" he yelled.

Most men don't want to admit that another man touched them sexually. Male survivors often fear that women will never look at them as men again, or they feel inferior to other men because of what happened. Even if they are gay, men rarely want to admit that they were forced. This construct shouldn't be ignored. Their reluctance has to be validated.

I said to him, "I know as a guy, you can't say anything. Basically, you can just be pissed off about it, I get that."

After a man discloses to me, there are a lot of things going on in the room. He is uncomfortable and at his most vulnerable. He is a raw nerve. That is when I validate his story with a comment like, "That's not your fault," or "You were just a kid, that's not OK." It sounds simple, but the point is that I've acknowledged and validated rather than dismissed his story.

When I go into prisons, I walk in with no fear – I have to; prisoners can smell fear. I treat them like human beings and equals. They have to call me Dr. Warner so I address them as Mr. along with their last name. I make sure we are on an even playing field at all times – I am no more and no less than they are. This allows me to get much farther with them than others.

As our relationship develops, my guys often call me their "protective spirit" or the "protective mother they never had." Many of these men had mothers or caregivers who did not protect them or did not listen to them when they tried to disclose. Their mothers said things like "Isn't that just boys being boys?" which is what my husband's mother told him. I get a chance to confront that pain and hopefully replace it with a different memory.

The great irony in this is that I am married to a male survivor. Despite my experience as a psychologist, I didn't have the slightest clue of how to handle this relationship, and no resources were available to me.

It's easy for me to walk into a prison and analyze society's most problematic cases in a matter of hours. But as soon as I met Robert, the subject was no longer a subject. I was no longer blessed by objectivity. The issue of male trauma affected me at my deepest personal level. Once brought to the surface, it was now in my home - a part of our lives. I needed answers and resources that were not available to me as a spouse.

This was the first time in my life I was unable to conjure up a solution when faced with a problem.

If you have picked up this book, you are probably looking for resources as well. That is my why. As one of few women working with male survivors and as the spouse of a male survivor, I am in a unique position to provide desperately needed resources. I was once as lost as you may feel right now even though I work in the field. So please understand that your state of confusion is normal and expected. I hope this book provides the missing pieces to the puzzle you are struggling to solve.

Even before I became immersed in male issues, I grew up around men that I looked up to and whose character is undeniably interwoven with mine. I was born in Fontana, California, with two wonderful, loving parents, three brothers, and a sister. I was very close to my father growing up – a true daddy's girl. My father was a drill sergeant in the military, and he kept things sewed up tight at home. My brothers had a different experience of our father than I did, and they seemed much closer to our mother. Don't get me wrong, I love my mother deeply, but I am a female version of my father. He and I did everything together.

We were your average middle-class American family. As a military family we socialized and hung around on the nearby base. The military in the 1970s was much more integrated than my small town of Fontana, so we were around all different types of people. I never thought too deeply about race or how it related to me, a black girl in a mostly white town.

But Fontana has its own dark history and racist roots. I remember shopping with my mother when we saw the local Klan chapter holding a protest over the hiring of a Hispanic man at a local bank. I asked my mother what it was all about. Without hesitating she responded, "Oh, they're dressed up for Halloween, honey, don't worry." As a child, that satisfied me until I later realized that we were shopping for Valentine's Day cards.

In first grade, I was the only black girl in my class and was asked to play Coretta Scott King in the school assembly. When I came home from school and told my mother, she went silent. She went to the local high school and had a drawing made of Coretta Scott King. She offered the solution that I could hold up a cutout of Coretta Scott King saying, "My daughter is not her, but will stand with pride to celebrate a great woman." That was the way my parents raised and protected us. They were strong people and showed me how to navigate racism and confront it head-on when I needed to – even if I had to do it alone.

There was one year in grammar school when boys came in crying on a weekly basis. I was always in tune with boys and knew that boys didn't – or weren't supposed to – cry in public. Everyone in my town worked in the steel mills, and I figured out their fathers were laid off as a result of an influx of Mexican immigrants who would do the same job for a lower wage. People did not understand the stress this placed on families. The father was stressed due to losing his job and likely fighting with the mother. In turn, the mother probably fought with the kids. There is no resolution because the job is lost, and the only thing any of them know is that someone different than them has taken their livelihood.

Even at that young age I was able to recognize that these young boys had no acceptable outlet to channel their behavior except for anger. Boys are conditioned from a young age that sadness isn't an acceptable emotion but anger is. The restriction placed on boys keeps them from expressing a full range of emotions; instead society tells them to express only anger. For some of the boys in my school and their families, this anger manifested as racism and xenophobia. Given freedom and encouragement to express emotions other than anger, those young boys could have been provided with a healthier way to cope. I learned to identify racism as a societal issue rather than a personal one. I never took any of it personally.

As one of the few black girls in school, this created an environment that left me pretty isolated growing up. The fact that I didn't get along with many of the girls, and wasn't into most girly things, made me even more painfully isolated.

Maybe it was my male-centric childhood that naturally pulled me towards men's issues; maybe it was fate, who knows. In either case, I have made this my life's work. After I married Robert and we had our son Lawrence, I felt a love that I had never known before. The three most important people in my life, two of them men – one of whom is a survivor – gave me the vision to provide education and awareness of male survivors with a renewed and more robust passion.

Love, vision, and passion. When these three qualities come together, we find a new strength and creativity that allows us to persevere and excel in any situation. Those emotions propelled my creation of the SCRIPT conference in 2015.

SCRIPT stands for the Summit on Community Resilience, Intervention, Prevention, and Training. The conference was designed with the intention of providing professionals with better tools for dealing with society's most pressing mental health issues. We bring together law enforcement agencies, psychologists, social workers, gang interventionists, nurses, and students from all around the world to address these issues on a local level. To date, we have trained and educated hundreds of professionals in ways of thinking and real-world applications that are at the forefront of innovation in providing care to our communities. Most importantly, it is free to the public. I have a goal of making education about male survivors as accessible to the general public as possible. What we are doing at SCRIPT and the resources I strive to provide were scarce for me, and so many others, for far too long. I want to end that. Our men, the people who love them, and society as a whole deserve tools to deal with male trauma.

If you are the spouse or partner of a male survivor you have heard things such as *you're just like the rest of them, you don't listen to me*, or *you'll never be able to understand.* These words are usually followed by silence or an abrupt exit (from either the room or the relationship) by the man. It's not my experience as a psychologist that taught me that; it's my experience as a wife.

The genesis for the SCRIPT conference was to get my husband's attention – to let him know that I hear him, understand him, and feel him. My friends and loved ones know I like to do everything big. So to get Robert's attention, I created an entire conference on male survivors.

The 2015 conference was such a success, and the topic of male survivors so well-received, that it became a yearly conference receiving corporate sponsorship. Additionally, we added speakers on crisis intervention, mental health issues and another issue on which I have worked substantially, gang intervention.

When I found out my husband was a male survivor, I sought out all the literature, studies, and lectures I could find on male survivors. That amounted to exactly one book that was written over 20 years ago. I ordered that book 11 years ago, and I am still waiting for it to be delivered! That is how scarce the information on this subject is. Even as a practicing psychologist I was in over my head when trying to deal with the effects of abuse in my own family. Most people who love a male survivor have no psychological training, and with so little information available, it is easy to feel alone in this journey.

In this book, I address topics from a professional viewpoint and from an everyday perspective. Together with top experts in the field, I identify the different kinds of trauma, how they look, and how their effects manifest in the survivor. Male survivor trauma is a unique male issue, and therefore interactions in marriages will be different than those stemming purely from normal male issues. Every man must deal with general issues in life such as getting older, losing testosterone, and even balding, but male survivor issues and the trauma that accompanies them are unique to this group. Before we can heal, we must understand that healing and education are synchronous.

Then we need to talk about you. Your experience as the spouse of a male survivor is different from that of other spouses. You've undoubtedly had crises of faith, anger at your spouse and his abuser, or issues with extended family that we will need to address. These are not the kind of issues we can put a Band-Aid on and pretend everything is OK. We have to bring these issues to the surface and confront them head on. We will work through the fear and pain and grow into a healthy place of security, compassion, and love.

Intimacy, romance issues, depression, self-esteem, self-help, self-care, and, of course, many questions regarding the children might be running through your head right now. If that made you as anxious to read as it made me to write, take a deep breath. We will cover all of those topics and together shine a spotlight directly into the dark, dusty attic of male trauma.

Chapter 2

His History

Robert A. Carey, Psy.D.

County of San Bernardino, California
Dept. of Mental Health

Guilt, shame, and humiliation have been my companions for most of my life. From the first time that I was exposed to sexual conduct, around age 4 or 5, I had an unexplainable feeling in my core that I had done something bad and I shouldn't talk about it. It was a source of angst and shame. My early exposure to sex severely distorted the normal development of relationship skills. As a preteen, my time was spent with someone much older than me who groomed me into abuse. I felt ashamed that I had been tricked. As a teen, a predator manipulated me to get back at her husband, and humiliation became part of my vocabulary.

The stage was set by parents who were young, dealing with their own issues, and not always paying attention to the right threats. I remember my mother always cleaning to the point that I just wanted her to stop cleaning and pay attention to me. I remember my father frequently distracted by beer and poker with his friends.

I label the sexual abuse of my childhood in chapters.

Chapter 1 – Guilt (age 4 or 5)

I was hanging out one day with a bunch of older kids when a game of truth or dare broke out in an upstairs bedroom. When it was my turn, I took the dare, which was performing a sexual act on a teenage girl. What happened isn't important – it's the feelings and thoughts afterward that had long-term effects. I was prodded and goaded to perform the dare, and this peer pressure taught me to listen to others and do what they told me.

I *knew* I wasn't supposed to talk about what just happened. I don't recall anyone saying I shouldn't talk about it, but there was a voice in my head saying that if I shared this, it would not be good. I felt guilt in a way that went to my core and has taken years of therapy to uncover and examine. My view of sex was warped at that point, and the guilt that surrounded it became the foundation for later abuses. I am not sure if the events of that day harmed me (I can't even clearly remember all of the details), but I know the stigma that became attached to anything sexual caused me years of needless suffering.

Chapter 2 – Shame (age 6 or 7)

When my parents divorced, I would spend every other weekend with my dad. He wasn't very good at taking care of himself, let alone caring for a child. He spent far too much time drinking and playing poker when he should have been looking after me. It's the same story as many abuse survivors – no one was paying attention so it was easy for the predator to manipulate the situation. With no adult supervision, someone who was twice my age had an easy time grooming me into having sex while I was way too young to consent with any real knowledge of what I was doing. This continued for about six years. By the time I put an end to the abuse, I was a preteen and he was almost an adult.

I felt shame about what happened, but even more, I was ashamed because of the way I was convinced to participate.

It was this manipulation of my consent, the mind games that did real damage to me. I was never forced into anything, but I was frequently tricked. That is where the long-term effects still play out today. I don't trust people when I first meet them. I am highly skeptical of other's motives until they are proven honest and ethical.

Chapter 3 – Humiliation (age 16)

I was a big kid. At 16, I was an impressive six feet tall and about 185 pounds, but I still felt small inside. This sense of myself as small made it easy for others to take advantage of me, even if they were physically smaller than me. I think because I had been groomed to do what others wanted from that first time of seeking female approval at 4 years old, it was easy for the abuse of Chapter 3 to happen.

Humiliation came to me in the form of a 28-year-old woman who was my aunt by marriage. With my history of being groomed, I was easy pickings to be a pawn in this predator's game.

At this time, both my parents were distracted with new relationships. I felt like I was asserting my independence, and I started living with my aunt and uncle. At first, she would come down at night and have sex with me while her husband slept upstairs. I was pretty drunk with the attention she was paying me and oblivious to the wrongness of the situation.

When reality hit and the damage was discovered, I remember my uncle saying to me, "If it was anybody else, I'd kill you." Looking back, I think he reacted that way because he realized I was just a kid. My mother's reaction was to treat me as an adult who had done something wrong.

Despite initial attempts to hush up the situation, the gossip eventually spread through the family. The humiliation I felt was the scar I bore for years afterward.

***

The inevitable result of having a history like mine is a detour into low self-esteem, drugs, alcohol, bad relationships, and dysfunctional coping skills. My first marriage was to a woman who was obsessed with my whereabouts and who I was with. She was convinced I was cheating on her even when I was at work in a store where every square inch was exposed to windows. The relationship was toxic on every level to the point where I seriously wondered if she was poisoning me when she said, "I'd watch what I eat around here if I were you. You never know what might be in the food."

I didn't know what or who to believe in life, but when she came along and was so attentive, I trusted her. It's what survivors do, and it's what makes them vulnerable to predator's tricks. When she said something, I simply believed it because I wanted to feel loved. If she said I was the reason that we weren't pregnant, it must be true. No need to check with a doctor!

Today my coping skills are better though they do not come naturally to me. I have to focus and work at not reacting right away. If I'm given time to reflect, I can come back to a situation with a calm, reasoned response.

Oftentimes I will "hide under the bed," as my wife Debra calls it. I need the time to tease out my feelings and think through what is real and what is not. Historically, I've been so manipulated, tricked and humiliated that I don't know what I'm feeling right away.

The inability to trust people, the discomfort around sex and relationships, my underdeveloped coping skills – these were (and still are to some degree) the long-term effects that Debra and I must contend with. It's not easy, but it's getting better.

Talking about what happened has taken away much of the guilt and shame. Learning to be open about sex and my feelings has been a process. It is for everyone. For survivors though, we have additional layers of protective scar tissue to work through.

Shedding the humiliation of my teens has taken years and many hours with therapists to see that my part in that drama was as a pawn, not a knight and certainly not a king.

That means I had limited moves and was easily sacrificed by the queen for her own survival. As a kid, I wasn't responsible for the situation. The humiliation belongs to the abuser, not to me.

In life, there is what happens to us and then what we learn from it. I carried around the harmful lessons I learned as a young child and then a young man for years. The emotional wounds and the mental scars are the effects of what happened and remain doing more harm until examined.

But my history, both the good and the bad, is what has made me who I am. Day by day, the wounds are healed, and I replace the pain of years gone by with love and the joy that I share with my wife and family.

Chapter 3

My Husband's Abuse

I would classify my husband's trauma as mid-range on the spectrum of severity. He would as well. Any trauma, whether it is emotional, physical, or sexual, has a significant impact on children, and influences much of the behavior that they will exhibit in future relationships.

Robert had several experiences of abuse that crossed all three categories – emotional, physical, and sexual. His abuse also consisted of multiple instances over the course of his childhood. One of those abusive relationships was incestuous.

Robert was first exposed to sexual activity when he was around 4 years old. Robert's parents divorced when he was 6 years old, and after that, he split his time between the two homes.

His abuser at the time of his parents' divorce was a 12-year-old kid we will call Sammy who lived down the street from Robert's father. Robert would sleep over at Sammy's house on the weekend, and it was during these sleepovers that he was abused.

Your instincts may be pointing at the glaring red flag of a 6-year-old child sleeping over a 12 year old's house. The age difference is significant and the children are at very different stages in their development. So, why would any parent in their right mind allow their 6-year-old son to sleep over at Sammy's house?

This is where the emotional trauma my husband endured sets the stage for future sexual abuse. His parents were preoccupied and distant when he was growing up. They weren't paying attention to risks involved when they allowed him to sleep at an older boy's house.

Robert had no way of knowing that this was not a normal encounter. At 6 years old, children aren't aware of what is normal and what is not. Becoming sexualized at this young age sounds crazy to any rational person, but a 6 year old doesn't know any better. Such behavior then becomes normal for him. Abuse victims are groomed to believe that the abuse is normal. Robert, like most childhood sexual trauma victims, was also groomed not to tell anyone what was going on.

Grooming is the process by which an abuser gains a child's trust and develops an emotional connection with them. In some cases, the abuser grooms the family and develops an emotional connection with them, as well. Part of the purpose for developing that trust is to ensure the child will keep a secret.

Abusers look for vulnerable or unsupervised children who they know will be left alone. A few years back, I heard a story on the car radio about a child who was found wandering around a Lego store in California. The child's parents had dropped him off and left him to check out the store on his own. According to store policy, an employee took the child into the back of the store and watched him until the parents picked him up. When they returned, they were upset with the employee for interrupting the child's time!

Listeners were invited to call in and voice their opinion. Most sided with the parents of the child. But what the Lego employee did was right, and that is a clever store policy to deter would-be abusers.

It is exactly such scenarios that pedophiles look for. A potential abuser seeing a child wandering alone around a store will observe that the child is unsupervised and try to befriend him. When the parents arrive, the abuser will befriend them, as well. The pedophile knows that eventually he will be able to groom the child and get him alone due to a lack of parental supervision.

An example of the grooming process may look like this: The abuser will give the kid candy and say something like, "I know your parents don't let you have candy. Take a piece, and don't tell them. It will be our secret." After a few weeks the same situation repeats itself only now instead of candy, it's cigarettes. The child knows they are doing something wrong, but a surface layer of trust has been established since the child didn't tell their parents about the candy last time. If the child keeps the secret about smoking a cigarette, then the process continues.

Next, the abuser may show the child pornography. The abuser will normalize the behavior to the child and ask if he is interested in trying what he is seeing. After a few weeks the abuser may put a hand on the child's leg, but nothing more, just to see if the child will keep a secret about that. This process will usually take place over the course of several weeks or months. At every stage of the grooming process, the child is being conditioned, coerced, and possibly threatened to keep the secrets. Threatening harm directly to the child or to the child's family are regular ploys used by the abuser to keep children isolated. The end result of the grooming process is some form of sexual abuse which the child is now conditioned, or groomed, to think is normal. This doesn't mean that the grooming process will end in penetration every time. It might not. But it can lead to sexual contact, and that can escalate to penetration as the child is further groomed over the course of weeks, months, or years.

Other forms of sexual abuse can result from the grooming process, for example, child pornography. The child may be conditioned to allow suggestive or sexual pictures to be taken of them. No matter the abuser's end goal, the patterns of gaining trust and access, while maintaining secrecy and isolation, are universal principles of the grooming process. The specifics will look different in each unique situation and with each abuser, depending on the type of sexual contact they are into and what they think they can get away with.

The notion that abuse abruptly occurs by force is a misconception. It most often occurs as the result of a grooming process and is a series of progressions. Throughout each stage, trust is being developed between the abuser and the victim. The abuser tricks the child into keeping secrets from their parents. The abuser draws them in, luring them at every subtle manipulation, and once the abuse takes place, the child fears telling anyone. They think they will be the ones who get in trouble. The grooming process perpetuates the abuse.

The abuser has to gain the trust of the parents in order to have access to the child, and will groom them as well. That is why cases in which the abuser is mom's boyfriend or dad's girlfriend are common. It is about access to the child, and with the built-in trust these positions garner, access is inherent.

The two biggest cases of serial pedophilia in recent memory are the Jerry Sandusky case and the scandal involving scores of Catholic priests. What did those situations have that is a common thread of many pedophilia cases? The abusers had unquestioned access to children, and were inherently trusted as a result of their positions.

Jerry Sandusky was an assistant football coach under head coach Joe Paterno at Pennsylvania State University. He founded the Second Mile, a non-profit that served underprivileged and at-risk youth. As a part of Second Mile, he hosted several youth football camps in the summer.

His non-profit, as well as his power and authority in the community, gave him full access to children, many of whom were vulnerable due to their economic circumstances. This vulnerability was used as a tool to exploit and silence the victims and perpetuate the abuse. No one dared to question

Sandusky because he was a high profile football coach at a national championship caliber program.

The scandals that plagued the Catholic Church were cut of a similar cloth. Priests have access to children through after school programs, religious activities, and charities. People within the community rarely suspect them of wrongdoing because they are seen as paragons of virtue and are revered as such.

Access to children and presumed trustworthiness are key to the positions that many pedophiles seek and hold in their community or family. They will abuse this level of trust and exploit the access it gives them to children.

My son Lawrence attends a Tae Kwon Do class with a group of roughly 50 other children ages 4 to 8. Their teacher Master Jon is adored by the students and parents alike. He holds a position of power that was not questioned.

During one of his classes, Lawrence had to get dressed into his gi, and Master Jon's wife took him in the bathroom to change. When I saw this happening, bells and flashing lights went off in my motherly antenna. I walked through the class and, in front of everyone in the studio, including parents, I opened the door to the bathroom and followed them in. I came out and my husband looked at me with a half-smile and said, "As soon as she did that, I knew exactly what you were going to do."

The look of shock and bewilderment on the faces of other parents showed that they thought I was crazy, but I didn't care – that is my son. One mistake I often see is that parents care too much about what people think of them. What parents need to keep in mind is that in 10 years it won't matter what those people thought of you. What will matter is the well-being of your child.

A few months later, I took Lawrence to class and Master Jon greeted him with a kiss on the cheek. Again, the whistles and lights were going off in my mommy brain. I thought that was very unusual, and by my standards it was downright weird so I made sure to come back the next week to see if it happened again.

I observed the same behavior the following week so I asked my son after class, "Do you like Master Jon?" "Yeah," he said, without giving it any thought and continuing to look at passing cars out the window. "Is he nice to you?" "Yeah," he again replied. "Good."

I filled my parents in on the situation, and asked them to come with me to the following class so they could observe for themselves. Maybe I was overreacting, so I figured it was a good idea to bring in an extra set of eyes. They thought that while it was a little bizarre, it appeared to be normal, and I may be making a bigger deal of it than it was. That was fine, I could accept that. But I was sure going to investigate. I would rather make a bigger deal out of nothing than fail in my due diligence as a parent to keep my child safe.

In the process of investigating and bringing my parents along for a second opinion, I was also increasing my visibility. Although I was remaining silent, I was being intimidating and assertive, and showing that I was more trouble than any grooming process would be worth. This was part of my strategy, too. Abusers pick the child that is paid the least attention or the one that no one will believe. The last thing they want to deal with are hawkish parents.

A week later I asked my son if Master Jon ever made him feel uncomfortable. Then a few weeks after that, I asked him if Master Jon ever made him do anything outside of Tae Kwon Do class. I spaced all of these questions weeks apart on purpose as to not alarm my son or create a fear inside of him that he otherwise would not have. All of those answers were "no's" to my satisfaction.

If you ever find yourself in a situation that sets off your parental alarm and you have to ask the same questions I asked my son, look for consistency in responses. If a child becomes embarrassed and runs away or exclaims "No!" and then runs away, something may be wrong, and it is worth investigating further. Teenagers especially do not want to discuss anything sexual with their parents, and may answer with a "no, that's gross," but later change details of their story. Anything out of the ordinary or inconsistent with your child's normal behavior is something you want to pay attention to.

Being available for your children is the best way to prevent grooming and subsequent abuse. Spend quality time with your kids, and listen to them. I meet a lot of parents who are always eager to drop off their child with friends or family so they can catch some well-deserved time for themselves. It is a normal part of life. But if your child starts saying things like, "I don't want to go there" every time you drop him off, that is a red flag. If your child tells you that someone makes them feel "creepy" or something similar, inquire further. Don't dismiss it. Robert's parents were not paying attention to the inconsistency in, and around, him.

Robert's earliest abuse took place when he was 4 or 5 years old by a group of kids between 12 and 13 years old. During a game of truth or dare, Robert was dared to perform a sexual act on one of the girls.

The sexual abuse with the teenage girl was significant for a few reasons all related to conditioning. For my husband, this conditioned a lack of control in sexual situations that essentially told him that he has no power of choice. This was also the first woman who abused him. I believe this created vulnerability to his aunt's later abuse because he now had the experience of not being in control in sexual situations with older women. The door to subsequent inappropriate behavior was open. The age appropriate boundaries of sexual exploration that were supposed to be present were ripped down by sexual abuse. They were violated and disintegrated. When his aunt seduced him, he had no reference point for boundaries. He had no power to say no. Robert did what all of us do – repeat the behaviors we learn throughout our lives.

There is a certain innocence and giddiness that comes with normal sexual exploration as a teenager. You flirt, then hold hands, and maybe after a couple of dates to the movies, you kiss. There is a process of exploration. This kind of innocence and process was gone for Robert. There were overt sexual acts instead of a natural process. There was no giddy innocence, but rather a secret wrongness to the relationship. Also, these acts were done to him rather than with him. They were brought on to him by force rather than through his willing participation. It was conditioned into Robert, as it is in many male survivors, that sex is something "dirty" or "bad" and must be kept secret.

Robert's third abuser was his aunt, who began molesting him at 16 years old. The abuse lasted for six to eight months. The abuser was so cunning that she convinced him to move into her home, where she lived with her husband and two kids, to continue the abuse. Robert's mother found out about the abuse, and years later said, "You just can't take sex away from a teenager." This was yet another dismissal, minimization, and additional emotional baggage that a young man had to unpack and sort out later in life. After this abuse, Robert tried to kill himself at the age of 16. Like so many others, he sought an end to the untreated emotional suffering he was going through. Robert slashed his wrists in front of his girlfriend. The girl's father took him to his aunt and uncle's house, and they drove him to the hospital.

This highlights a theme I've seen in many men where multiple cases of abuse are present. There tends to be a dysfunction in the childhood environment that acts as an incubator for abuse. Parents, who are not present for their children as a result of factors like addiction, mental illness, or neglect, create environments in which abuse is more likely to occur.

Whenever news of something horrific emerges, what does everyone always say? *I never suspected anything. He was never the type to do that. He was always so nice.* Abusers are hardly going to announce, "Here I am!" nor do they wear a scarlet letter. They blend into society. They look like you and me. The same goes for victims. Often they do not tell anyone what they have experienced. Many survivors carry their secret to the grave.

For every known victim of a pedophile, there are more that are unknown. We find out this information from first-time offenders who get charged with sexual assault on a minor. They typically want a deal for a lighter sentence from the district attorney, and so they confess to other assaults in the hope that their cooperation will cast them in a more favorable light. I recently sat down with a prisoner who was convicted of a sex crime on a minor for the first time. He divulged to me other fantasies he had and the fact that he had acted out some of them, but he'd never been caught. Offenders like these are typical and frequently pass through the criminal justice system. Unfortunately, we do not find out about them until they commit a crime and are arrested.

Many victims go through life with few overt but many subtle signs of their abuse. For example, instead of obvious emotional outbursts, the straight-A student begins flunking out of school. They start using drugs. That is my husband's story. He attended a good private school and was a smart and athletic student. After the abuse with his aunt started in mid-adolescence, his life was thrown into turmoil. He flunked out of the private school, transferred to the local public high school, and got into drugs. I believe that his life took a turn down a much rougher road than he would have traveled had the abuse not occurred.

Abusers walk a dark path as well, hiding in the shadows that our culture provides them. The toughest pill to swallow for us as a society is the fact that our culture fosters and perpetuates the abuse of male victims. We unknowingly provide shelter for abusers with our societal norms for masculinity.

Our society blames male victims of sexual abuse more harshly than any other victim demographic. We have been accustomed to believing that men cannot be raped - they can only rape. If a man comes forward with his story of abuse, he is silenced, shunned, and dismissed. This can create additional and exacerbated trauma. Equally as upsetting and prevalent is when the male victim has a female abuser and is told "you should be happy that you got laid."

The general population is accustomed to a certain cultural norm regarding masculinity. While the gender expectations for women have radically changed in the last 50 years, the concept of masculinity has remained almost as rigid as it was a century ago. Men are supposed to be strong independent and devoid of emotions considered "feminine" such as sadness and anxiety. Men are typically told to "suck it up" and stop complaining.

What kind of message does this send to male victims of sexual trauma? It tells them that they are not important, and they are not heard. If a man rapes another man, many times the victim is told he "should've pushed the guy off of him."

It is the contrary if a woman rapes a man. That man is told that he should've liked it or that men cannot be raped. These types of responses, which are pervasive in our society, provide the cultural blind spots that abusers hide in. That is why so many male victims keep silent about their abuse.

Many of the fights I have had with Robert have been the result of his feeling that I did not hear him. As the spouse of a survivor, you can probably relate to that. They feel that no one hears them, and they have no voice. It creates a massive chip on their shoulders that often plays out in relationships with them feeling on the defensive. It is a common theme among male survivors, and it is directly tied to the culture we have created based on antiquated ideas of masculinity and male sexuality.

Society's idea of masculinity – not verbalizing emotion, "sucking it up," and the need for a large sexual appetite – can make men feel inferior. Those stigmas can add to the pressure that a male survivor already feels and force him to keep his silence.

There may have been a time in the past when the male survivor you love disclosed to someone and received a dismissive or belittling response. Maybe they decided they would never tell anyone again. This wall of silence, and the idea of what a man should be, keeps many survivors from disclosing their secret to anyone, especially their spouse. The culmination of these toxic factors led Robert to an early suicide attempt, decades of silence, and plenty of wreckage in his life that was related to unresolved trauma.

When I work in prison populations, sometimes I am lucky enough to be the person who crosses paths with a survivor during that crucial, once-in-a-lifetime window of opportunity where they are ready to disclose. When I am face-to-face with a man who is a survivor and he begins to leak parts of his story, all I have to do is sit and listen. There are no special words that need to be said. On the contrary, anything I say could be the trigger that sends him back into his shell with his secret retreating into the dark.

This man may have tried to disclose numerous times before only to be met with whatever projection of societal norm the receiver put forth. I sit in silence and let him drip until the dam breaks and the secret comes pouring out. This doesn't take any special training or degrees, just the willingness to listen. Listen with compassion and understanding. Don't interrupt a survivor in the middle of a disclosure, and thank him for disclosing to you when he is finished. A whole new dimension of your relationship will open, and an entire field of interpersonal growth will flower and become available for both of you.

Chapter 4

Types of Abusers

Before we go forward, we need to agree on the definitions of abuse and trauma. There are so many definitions and nuances of both that it can be easy for people to misunderstand one another. For our purposes, I prefer using the word "trauma" over "abuse."

Trauma can be any event or the witnessing of an event that causes a great deal of distress. Trauma encompasses everything from being the victim of an assault or sexual abuse to witnessing someone else being assaulted. All of these potential distresses are covered under the umbrella of trauma.

Abuse implies another person performed an action to you that distressed you. From my perspective, this definition is limited in its scope, and therefore I prefer using the overarching, more encompassing definition of trauma. For the purpose of this book, trauma can be applied in a more accurate fashion than the word abuse. However, when referring to specific cases of trauma that include physical actions such as assault, the word abuse will be used as it allows for specificity.

Abusers can be divided into two categories under which other subsets exist: pedophiles and hebephiles. Pedophiles are sexually attracted to prepubescent children while hebephiles are attracted to children who have begun puberty. The abusive treatment and patterns can be very similar. The main difference is in the physical appearance of the children they seek. Hebephiles prefer children generally aged between 11 and 14 who have more matured bodies with some adult characteristics. Pedophiles are attracted to prepubescent children who do not possess an adult body shape.

My husband was sexually abused by both categories of abusers. When he was 6 years old, his abuser was a pedophile; his abuser at 16 years of age was a hebephile. It is a common misconception that only adults can be pedophiles. Teenagers, such as Sammy, can also be pedophiles.

Pedophilia is an innate tendency that is hardwired into the brain. While pedophiles can curb their tendencies and take preventive measures to keep themselves from acting out like avoiding high-risk situations, they will always have an innate attraction to children.

The attraction to children specifically stems from the innocence of childhood. Many pedophiles are attracted to that innocence and the taking of that innocence, and find these concepts erotic.

There is a misconception called the "vampire myth" that I will mention here briefly, but it is addressed later at length in its own chapter. The "vampire myth" states that a person who is molested as a child has a greater likelihood of becoming an abuser later in life. This claim is based on studies of people who were incarcerated for sexual abuse crimes, thus creating biased and skewed results. Studies using data from the general population have discredited the vampire myth.

While pedophilia is an innate tendency hardwired into the brain, it can be behaviorally modified by avoiding people, places, and things that are known triggers. Approaches such as cognitive behavioral therapy are effective at getting a pedophile to see their triggers and avoid them. The key is the pedophile has to want to change, but many times they don't believe what they are doing is wrong. They believe society is wrong or that society doesn't accept them for who they are.

When I interview a pedophile or rapist, I have to first establish that I am not judging them. If I don't establish a safe and non-judgmental space, then I won't get the information I need from them. When I work with pedophiles, one of the exercises I conduct makes them recall backwards from the moment they abused a child. I ask them to recall one minute before the abuse, and one minute before that, and I do this to find the ritual and triggers in their abuse. Once we find this information, we can work on changing it. As a clinician, this information is also crucial to understanding their psyche and makes me better at my job.

Within the classification of pedophiles, there are three subsets that generally describe the characteristics that pedophiles prefer in a victim: regressed, fixed, and mixed.

A regressed pedophile or hebephile believes the child they are molesting is the same age as they are. They believe the child is mature enough to desire and therefore consent to a sexual or intimate relationship with them. They regress and bring the child up to their age, thus the term "regressed." They also find pleasure in the belief that they are showing an innocent child the ways of the world. While working with regressed pedophiles and hebephiles in prison populations, I have heard them say statements like *She seduced me* or *She wanted it.* Some even bought the child wedding clothes believing the child to be mature enough to marry them.

Fixed pedophiles prefer a specific age range, for example 6- to 11-year-old children. They seek victims within their preferred range and when the child outgrows the age, they discard them and look for a new victim. Fixed pedophiles also prefer a certain type of look. This can be specified by race, hair color, clothing preference, or any number of attributes that relates to a "look" someone has. I have seen in fixed pedophiles that were molested as children, some aspect of trying to reclaim or being attracted to the childhood that was lost for them. In this group, the pedophile is usually fixed on the age at which he or she was molested.

Mixed pedophiles have a combination of both classifications. They may prefer a certain look or age range, but also may believe a child is functioning at the same cognitive level they are. Mixed pedophilia combines the physical characteristics that a fixed pedophile desires, but with the cognitive functioning that a regressed pedophile believes a child is operating at.

Pedophiles and hebephiles can also be classified with rapists. Most rapists act out sexual abuse that can be classified into power-control, sadistic, and ritualistic categories by certain characteristics. The power-control abuser is feeling powerful and superior to the victim. This is the most common type of rapist, and abuse typically tends to orbit the power-control dynamic. Power-control abusers don't want consent. Instead, they want the victim to fight so they can overpower them and be given the feeling that they have taken something from the victim. Most sexual abuse has a power-control dynamic to it. Over the years, I have talked to thousands of rapists and pedophiles, and in many of their crimes the desire and presence of control was a primary element.

Sadistic abuse is centered on inflicting pain and hurting the victim. There is a power-control dynamic at play in sadistic abuse as well, as the abuser holds the power to inflict pain on the victim.

One of my early cases was a sadistic-hebephile rapist I will call John. John and an accomplice kidnapped a 14-year-old girl who was a mutual acquaintance. They forced her into a van and while the accomplice drove, John tied her up and began to rape and beat her. John was so violent that he ripped the girl's breast off her body during the course of the sexual and physical assault. This was a sadistic rape with the intention of inflicting major pain on the victim.

Ritualistic abuse has a ritual or ceremony behind the act that is sometimes but not always religious in nature. The pattern may be that the abuser has to tie up their victim or they have to torture them until they beg for their life. Some rapists will bleed or maim their victims because they believe God will purify them. The ritual looks very different in each case of abuse, but completion of it in the correct way is necessary for a ritualistic abuser to achieve satisfaction. It is like a craving or an appetite that they have to satisfy.

The child abuser seeks control of the relationship and the child. Physically, the abuser is probably much larger than the victim. This size difference between the abuser and victim creates a psychological trauma. A typical response to this psychological factor is that male survivors are unaware of their size in adulthood. They always feel like they have to prove they are bigger than everyone else, and therefore physically secure.

Robert is 6 feet tall and weighs 300 pounds. He played football growing up and still looks like he could be a lineman on a professional football team. He is a large, powerful man. But he is unaware of this fact and thinks he is physically small in stature. In response, he carries a chip on his shoulder with the desire to prove he is physically bigger than everyone else by puffing out his chest and standing up straight. This may be flattering to him but intimidating to others. Most of the time, he is already the biggest guy in the room. There is no need to prove his size to anyone. For the survivor, an idea of physical inferiority is deeply rooted in his psyche as a result of childhood abuse and the physical difference in the size of their abuser.

Abuse can be classified as emotional, physical, or sexual, but few cases fit entirely into one category. Rather most contain elements of two or more categories.

For the purpose of this book, it is necessary we identify the other types of abuse that affect human relations. Physical abuse is intentional contact which causes trauma, such as punching, slapping, or kicking. A child growing up in a violent household is always walking on eggshells. They don't know when the next blow up is going to happen or what it is they might do that will cause it. Constantly wondering when the other shoe is going to drop, they are always on guard and doing their best not to be the target of violence.

Imagine being a 5-year-old child living in an alcoholic household where one parent routinely comes home drunk and beats the other parent. At that young age, the cognitive ability cannot fully understand the factors at play: the disease of addiction, domestic violence cycles, and mental health issues. Instead, the house is a battleground, and the violence is random and unpredictable.

This child has no security in his or her home and is simply focused on surviving. A survival technique typical of a small child is hiding under the bed. When they hear mom or dad coming home late at night from the bar and the sound of household items breaking, they hide under the bed and from the violence outside the bedroom.

Coping mechanisms that work for us as children tend to be our default ones as adults. For the survivor of physical abuse, "hiding under the bed," as I have come to label it, is a carryover of this coping behavior. Think back to times when you and your significant other got into an argument or when there was tension building up to an argument. Out of nowhere they may decide to go on a fishing trip for two weeks or they leave home and don't answer texts or calls for several days. It is as if they pull a disappearing act at the first sign of conflict, even though there is no threat of physical violence. Their brains are hardwired to avoid conflict by acting out in this manner through this behavior. For the spouses, the behavior seems insane; we can't begin to understand it. We start wondering: Where is he? Who is he with? Who is *she*?

When Robert and I were in the early stages of our relationship, we were living in a small, rural town outside Chicago. It was a typical Midwestern setting with one main street and a single stop light. The whole town looked like it was carved out of the large cornfield that surrounded it.

I was in graduate school at the time, and during one of the breaks we planned a vacation. As part of our preparations, we had to go to the bank and withdraw money for the trip.

At the bank, we found that Robert had made a mistake with our finances through an accounting error, and we were out $300. To a couple of students living paycheck to paycheck, this was a lot of money to lose. On the ride home, I was visibly and verbally upset. "We can't be doing this, that's a lot of money," I said. Robert lost it at that comment. He took it as if I was attacking who he was fundamentally as a person. But rather than yelling, he waited until we stopped at a light, then he opened the car door, sprinted across the street, and disappeared. We were at least 30 miles from home. I spent nearly 20 minutes looking for him to no avail. I was in utter disbelief, so I let it be. After some time, Robert emerged, seemingly out of thin air, and got back in the car. We drove home in silence. I didn't ridicule him or flip out. I knew he had been "hiding under the bed."

Survivors of trauma – especially physical abuse – have a very difficult time connecting with other people, and often sabotage friendships and relationships.

As children, failing to meet expectations resulted in violence. For example, if they did poorly in school, they were hit. If they dropped a touchdown in the football game, they were told how much of a disappointment they were. The situations are varied, but the common theme is that violence was used when expectations were not met. For most children, mistakes are learning opportunities, but for survivors they were a source of terror as abuse usually followed.

As adult survivors, on a subconscious level, life becomes all about avoiding the violence that they experienced as children. They strive to be the best, and they are reluctant to accept or seek help because in their minds that is synonymous with weakness. When they make a mistake or feel tension building, the most familiar tool they have is to push away - to be totally alone. If they are alone, there is no one to let down and no violence to suffer through. The survivor pushes people away and builds walls a mile high and does so subconsciously, unaware of what they are doing and why. Spouses tend to internalize this behavior rather than confronting it head on, because it will keep the peace in the home or they don't want to make the situation worse.

When sexual abuse is a part of the survivor's story, passion and sex are severed from one another. Love looks very different than a non-survivor's conception of it. It lacks sexual and physical contact. When engaged in any sort of sexual activity, the survivor can seem devoid of emotion and sex can become mechanical. A male survivor of sexual trauma has been conditioned into thinking sex is something bad. I have spoken to thousands of survivors over the years and they tend to describe themselves as two things: bad and dirty. Those are the two words that come to mind for most survivors when they are talking about themselves in relation to sex. It is tough to reverse that kind of conditioning towards sex, but it is possible.

Sex and intimacy is something that has to be explored between you and your husband. I talk to couples about this frequently and encourage them to go to couples counseling in order to improve their sex lives. I'm usually met with pushback about how uncomfortable it is to talk to a total stranger about problems in the bedroom. It is uncomfortable, but most couples come back to me after a period of time and thank me for saving their marriage. As a spouse, our tendency is to think there is something wrong with us – either we are not attractive or good enough. That is not true, and therapy will help you see the error in that way of thinking. It took me years to figure out that I was not the reason for the issues Robert and I had regarding sex. I hope that you don't have to suffer with those self-destructive thoughts as long as I chose to.

Emotional trauma can be associated with physical or sexual trauma or it may occur on its own. For the male survivor, few people are trustworthy or consistent. Survivors may trust others to a certain extent, but rarely will they let others take a peek into the deep, shadowed recesses of their heart and soul. That is a forbidden place that few, if any, will see. When I first started talking to my husband during the normal courting process, the conversation would always skip over his childhood. I would ask him what it was like, and I would get a bland generic response like *It was a normal childhood.* He wasn't ready to let me see what was behind that door. Survivors keep people, especially their spouses, at an arm's length, and are very careful not to give away too much information, if any at all. Many spouses believe this is an indictment of them, that they aren't worthy or good enough to be trusted with this information. That is not the case, and really it has nothing to do with the spouse at all. The survivor's feelings of guilt, shame, and inadequacy towards themselves can keep them closed off from others.

Gender of the abuser does play a factor in how the abuse affects a male survivor. Male-on-male abuse burdens the survivor with a deep societal shame, based on our ideas of what masculinity is. For a man, admitting that another man sexually abused him is shameful because it emasculates him. Much of society still erroneously believes that men cannot be raped.

When there is anal penetration involved, the abuse is much more damaging to the psyche. Forcibly being penetrated by another male creates a huge well of shame for the survivor. If penetration occurs, the long-term effects of abuse usually manifest much more intensely, both socially and emotionally, than abuse from kissing, fondling, or even oral sex. The trauma and the issues associated with that trauma, tend to interfere and disturb the male survivor's life to a much greater degree in cases of anal penetration.

Our culture reinforces this trauma by telling male victims that they should have done something to prevent the abuse. Men are supposed to be strong, and allowing another man to violate them in that way is seen as a glaring weakness or latent homosexuality. Male-on-male rape affects the psyche in a way that creates feelings of toxic shame as a "failure" or "inferior male" which will likely manifest in one of many ways: distancing relationships or avoiding them, sexual dysfunction, or not fulfilling potential and lack of success in life. Reginaldo Chase Espinoza, Psy. D. discusses this further:

"When a man believes he has failed to protect himself or 'rise above' a painful event, he takes undue responsibility for the tragedy. Perceived failure to protect is among the most impactful injuries to the male psyche. The fear of and belief that one has been inadequate in protecting himself or others is one of the leading reasons that men struggle to disclose victimization experiences (Tener & Murphy, 2015).

Men who take on irrational blame for their traumas can turn their anger inward toward the self, which may result in self-destructive patterns and a lifetime of punishment in their own minds. The male survivor may also carry tremendous anger toward his abuser(s), which can be misdirected if the anger is not effectively processed. Displaced anger can be directed at anyone who represents a threat or undermines the survivor's self-determination or ability to self-preserve. Much of the misdirection and dysregulation of anger is influenced by society's construction of masculinity, which must be challenged during the survivor's recovery and self-actualization processes after the abuse."

Males are also much more likely to admit a female abuser molested them because society's standards dictate that sex with a woman is something a man is supposed to be doing. Many times, male survivors of female-on-male abuse don't even internalize the fact that they've been raped. They may even deny that it was rape. When a boy is forced into having sex with a woman, it affects how that trauma manifests, causing sexual intimacy problems. The male survivor correlates sex with something that is wrong.

Female predators create psychological damage that differs from male abusers. This is a result of the things the women say while they abuse boys. For men sex is typically more of a physical act than it is for women, who tend to verbalize emotions during sex. Men have told me that the women who abused them said things like *I know you wanted me you remind me of your father, you're more of a man than my husband,* or make comments about the size of their penis.

Comments like these emotionally scar a young male in such a way that typically does not occur with a male predator. The result of this kind of systematic psychological abuse is emasculating to a young man, as they are being made to feel inferior, sub-human, or weak.

There can also be significant gender discrimination for male survivors of female abusers. I have worked with many survivors who possess a firmly rooted dislike of women, which is an outgrowth of the abuse they suffered as children.

Female predators have a tendency to mask their abuse behind a veil of being nurturing or motherly. As a society we don't look for female predators because no one suspects women to behave in this way. It is either too hard or uncomfortable for us to believe that a motherly figure could be capable of abusing a child. The reaction we have at a female taking a screaming child into a bathroom is much different than the reaction towards a male doing so. We are much more suspicious of the male's motives. We may even go so far as to question whether the child is really his. These kinds of suspicions are rarely raised towards females, who almost always get the benefit of the doubt. This is something that society allows to happen.

Abusers – regardless of gender – look for access to children. Many female abusers who have been in the news the past few years have been teachers. Just like the priest and football coach, the teacher is in a position of trust that gives her unquestioned access to children.

When the abuser is someone who is supposed to be taking care of you, such as a family member, a love/hate relationship called disorganized attachment occurs. For example, imagine the abuser is your father. You love your father and you always will. There is no conscious choice in the matter because he is the one who provides food and shelter for you. But you also hate your father because he is the source of abuse.

Gender roles as society defines them declare men the protectors and women the nurturers. When a child is abused, these gender norms are violated to the child. Women are no longer nurturing and men are the opposite of protectors so the child grows up lost. They have been betrayed by the people around them and have no sense of security. The motherly and fatherly roles have failed them.

A family dynamic plays out in homes that have sexual abuse occurring inside them, similar to the kind of dynamics that are at play in an alcoholic household – cycles of abuse, normalization, and the abuse becomes a family secret. As with an alcoholic family, a victim of the abuse will have to be the one who breaks the cycle for the generations that follow.

Robert's abuse came in cycles at ages 4, 6, and then at 16 by a family member. For his aunt, it was a normal way of sexualizing a teenage boy. The grooming process and subsequent abuse, conditions the child to thinking that this inappropriate behavior is normal.

Abuse of any kind – not just sexual abuse – can become a cultural norm. When we have a lack of diversity in our environment, we tend to see what is around us as normal. I always use the example of the turnip farmer. There is a turnip farmer who grows turnips in a small, rural town in the middle of America. He is taught how to farm his crops, as well as certain cultural norms. He has been taught that these are the keys to a happy life. His worldview is structured by the values of the culture he has grown up in. One day the turnip farmer is plucked from his plot of land in rural America and dropped in the middle of Times Square, New York City. What is he thinking? He is in complete culture shock. He has never seen anything like it. The city is sprawling with buildings that stretch into the sky. The people and their mannerisms are much different than the people he grew up around. Naturally, it is an insane scene to him. It is so radically different than what he has grown up around.

If all someone knows is abuse because that is what they have been raised with, then that person will grow up to believe their experience is normal. That is their world view, and they've been indoctrinated from a young age to believe it is the correct view. They are also conditioned not to trust anyone outside of the family because outsiders don't understand their way of life or cultural norms. They are told to never divulge the secrets of the family – namely the abuse – because outsiders won't understand. The result is the cycle of abuse perpetuating itself. The individual will keep living out the norms they have been taught.

It takes someone in the family to question the indoctrination, to rebel against the cultural norms, and break the cycle. My mother was raised in an alcoholic family in Texas and was surrounded by violence growing up. Her mother and aunt tried to kill someone with an axe due to domestic violence. Everyone in the family thought this kind of behavior was normal and they carried on with it, perpetuating it throughout generations until it came to an end with my mother. She saw the craziness around her and left the family. She married my father, and they left for California shortly after.

This same scenario carries out in families of abuse. Sexual abuse becomes a norm. In rare cases, the children are abused and groomed to be abusers themselves when they reach a certain age. However, most survivors break the cycle of abuse and do not go on to repeat the same traumatic behavior they endured.

Chapter 5

Manifestations of Trauma

Trauma refers to any situation or event that happened in the past which affects your present growth. Trauma can affect a person's social, cultural, and emotional functioning and can prevent them from engaging in activities of personal development.

Trauma isn't just damaging to the romantic relationship between you and your spouse; it is damaging across the lifespan of the male survivor. The traumatizing event becomes the defining story of the survivor's life, and all other relationships get caught up in the emotional entanglement that the trauma creates.

If the survivor has not yet dealt with his past, a multitude of issues, including financial, sexual, and physical, are impacted by the trauma, but the survivor is completely unaware of this impact.

This defining force in the lives of survivors drives how they pick their significant others. They often choose someone similar to them, as an alcoholic will find another alcoholic. They know what that person brings to the relationship because it is a similar trauma or pain. A survivor could go the opposite way and pick someone who is totally different from them - as the saying goes, opposites attract – because they think that person will be able to fix them. Women are rarely able to change significant others. He is what he is when he meets you, even though he may be driven subconsciously to find someone who can fix him. I know intuitively that my husband found me because he thought I could fix him or help him navigate his past.

Before we were together, he was married to another woman for 15 years who couldn't fix him, and I can't either. I have never tried to change my husband, and I don't try to change any of the survivors I work with. I allow them their space to work through their issues themselves. I accept them for who they are, and set my own boundaries.

With a male survivor, the concept of bonding with another human is distorted whether in a romantic or other relationship. The way a male survivor attaches to a spouse and the value system he brings to a relationship have been significantly shaped by the abuse. Reginaldo Chase Espinoza, Psy.D. talks about this further:

"Survivors may hold distorted views of bonding and abuse, due to historical betrayals that resulted in trauma (Alaggia & Ramona, 2014). These men, particularly with multiple betrayal traumas, may have associated betrayal and abuse with normative close relationships (Gobin, 2011). As a result, abuse may be somewhat expected, and loyalty and trustworthiness may not be actively sought after or a part of one's value system in relationships (Gobin, 2011). In such cases, survivors may experience several abusive relationships as an adult.

"Trauma bonding is a term used to describe the role of intense stress and fear in strengthening feelings of connection toward another. Attachment to another can intensify when self-identity is defined by the relationship, even when the expense is tremendous. Trauma bonding mostly occurs among individuals with low self-esteem, fear of not finding someone to care for or love them, and a heavy pattern of self-blame for their suffering (Katz, Arias, & Beach, 2000). The negative function of trauma bonding serves to keep a person in a relationship with a partner who causes or is associated with traumatic events."

As humans, we play out the trauma from our parents and childhoods in our first few relationships. It typically isn't until our third or fourth relationship that we start to get things right. Robert's first wife had not dealt with her trauma, just as Robert had not dealt with his. They sought each other on some unconscious level. Over the course of 15 years, they played out much of their trauma with each other. Robert endured abuse that almost cost him his life at the end of their relationship, as she was threatening to poison his food, telling him he "should watch what he eats around here." Dr. Espinoza also states:

"Especially among men with histories of childhood abuse, a fractured self-concept can bring about vulnerabilities that are difficult to communicate, tolerate, and change. Many victims internalize abuse and explain it as being related to fault, deserving punishment, weakness, or brokenness. (Draucker et al., 2009)."

This kind of relationship with a sadistic partner is well outside the realm of normal for someone who does not have a history of abuse, but for the survivor, this can be normal. Since the relationship with the abuser is inherently unequal with the abuser holding a position of power over the survivor, this creates fundamental feelings of inferiority and low self-worth, which are familiar and therefore comfortable despite being unhealthy.

As the child grows up, he doesn't know what it's like to be in a relationship where he is equal to his partner. He will perpetuate the fundamental belief of inferiority by seeking out sadistic and unhealthy relationships or partners to whom he can defer power, like the one Robert had with his first wife.

If emotional abuse is present, which it almost always is if other forms of abuse occurred, the survivor manifests these feelings of inferiority by becoming co-dependent to their partner. The desire of a child to receive a parent's love and positive attention is equal to the desire of food and water. It is a necessity. When they don't receive parental affection or receive negative attention, they search for it in romantic partners throughout their lives.

I have noticed a pattern in Robert, which I have seen in many other survivors. He does not want to feel like he is being blamed. This complex comes from the belief that the abuse was their fault. The abuser, as a form of grooming, could have pushed this belief on them, or it could be one they created within themselves. There are many times when Robert doesn't want to take ownership if things go wrong.

Making big decisions such as buying a house or car, or the household finances is a source of anger for Robert. As spouses we can enable this by taking over the family finances or making decisions on the next car or house to buy. Of course every person is unique, and this may manifest differently in your man, but I have found that a similar thread runs through the fabric of most male survivors.

I have traded the fact that I am enabling an unhealthy coping mechanism for a smoother running household. Sometimes it's necessary to make compromises like this to improve the functioning of the family system, but no one should be a doormat. In any marriage it takes a certain finesse to figure out where to give and take.

I met Robert six months after he and his wife separated. As I believe Robert's search to find someone who could help him with his trauma led him to me, I also believe his desire to help others with their trauma led him to the three wonderful girls he adopted, who are survivors of abuse as well. Robert possesses a piece of each of his daughters' pain, and as a whole they represent the sum of all of Robert's pain. When I married him, I also married those girls.

A common trait of survivors is trying to fix themselves through fixing other people. Certain events can trigger a survivor and send them in a neurotic tailspin of once dormant emotions. The birth of a child is one of these triggering events. When Robert and I had our son Lawrence, emotions surfaced in Robert that I had never seen in our relationship. He had anxiety that bordered on paranoia that Lawrence would have the same kind of childhood he did. He was always on edge and emotional blowouts were frequent in our house.

Routine issues that parents work through became heated arguments. Sometimes the attacks felt very personal in nature, and as a spouse this is how it often comes across. But I know that my husband is reacting from a place of fear and trauma that was untapped and not dealt with.

Emotional blowups like this can seem immature or even childish. When Robert would yell, he was like a 16 year old throwing a tantrum. I had never seen this flavor of anger from him before. The emotions that Lawrence's birth stirred up in Robert were coming from that damaged 16-year-old boy. Male survivors will lash out in ways typical of the emotional age of when the trauma happened.

The blowups came to a head one day when Robert was dropping me off at the beauty salon. We were looking for parking and I pointed out a spot, which he took as an attack on his driving. He began yelling in such a way that it seemed like his inner teenager took over. "You always do that! You don't listen!" he said. That proved to be the proverbial last straw for me. He needed to deal with his trauma or I was going to leave.

This is our story. Every survivor has their own unique story, yet many commonalities exist among those with traumatic histories of abuse. These commonalities include a variety of specific needs and consequences that must be addressed in many areas of survivors' lives. Dr. Espinoza discusses this point further:

"A large proportion of male survivors have acute and/or multiple traumas, which are often associated with varying degrees of traumatic stress. Traumatic stress responses can have many distinct dimensions, and not all survivors experience the same symptoms. Re-experiencing symptoms involves the triggering of intense situational fears, panic, and unsafe feelings, even including flashbacks to experiences of abuse. Avoidant symptoms involve intentional avoidance of thoughts, feelings, people, and situations related to traumatic events. Arousal symptoms involve hijacking of the brain, in which the survivor is periodically or persistently in a state of hypervigilance, due to a deep need to protect himself from potential threats. Dissociative symptoms involve a sort of psychological retreat, during which the survivor disconnects from surroundings, others, and even self. Numbness, low responsiveness, poor contact with reality, and reliance on fantasy can take hold of the survivor's mental processes.

"Male survivors experience a higher rate of psychiatric disorders than men without histories of abuse (Sparato, Mullen, Burgess, Wells, & Moss, 2004). Men with histories of abuse are also more likely to be victimized in adulthood, compared to men without such histories (Desai, Arias, Thompson, & Basile, 2002). Suicidal thoughts, post-traumatic stress disorder, chronic anxiety, and depression are among the leading mental illnesses among male survivors (George & Yarwood, 2004; Romano & De Luca, 2001). Loss of confidence, self-esteem, mistrust of others, guilt, shame, fear, feelings of brokenness, and confusion are frequent consequences of abuse that can persist until intentional healing is embarked upon (Mejia, 2005; George & Yarwood, 2004). These conditions and consequences can be reduced and managed over time, especially with the help of key resources such as psychotherapy and pharmacotherapy.

"Hurt, powerlessness, and threats can be reacted to for several years, even a lifetime, after surviving abuse (Draucker et al., 2009). In men, such experiences may be responded to with aggression and anger. Men with traumatic experiences of inescapable vulnerability may feel safer when transforming vulnerable emotions into anger. They may find that a mask of insensitivity can keep vulnerability and feelings of hurt at a predictable distance. Some male survivors may use learned aggressive behaviors as a method of exercising power and control to ward off potential threats and situational 'weakness.' Much of the anger is understandable, and certainly with merit, such as anger toward an abuser or close persons who failed to protect the survivor from abuse. However, anger may become more far reaching, and apparent in ways and situations that are inappropriate."

Survivors may use mind-altering substances, including alcohol, illicit drugs, and prescription medications, to suppress many of the problems resulting from the history of abuse. Trauma survivors, in fact, have one of the highest rates of substance abuse of any population with psychological issues. For loved ones and romantic partners, substance use can add a layer of complexity, concern, and obstacles to the relationship.

Substance abuse is not the only addictive or abnormally consuming behavior that can result from abuse-related distress. Some turn to food as a means of medicating their pain and discomfort. It's no coincidence that obesity rates are much higher among male and female survivors than in the general population. A larger body mass creates a sort of "safe space," a physical barrier between them and others. In their mind, their size protects them from abuse, either because others will not desire them or because they are much larger than the abuser.

Some may excessively focus on work or other activities that can cause a buildup of stress. Other survivors may develop obsessive-compulsive tendencies as a compensatory response to the loss of control experienced during and after abuse. Behavioral addictions are a symptom of a deeper problem, such as an inability to manage intense emotions or a lack of self-love. Thus, they should be viewed from a place of empathy and patience. Some addictions also may bring a fearsome host of behaviors, including financial irresponsibility, gambling, and not taking responsibility for actions. Acting out sexually is another common manifestation that occurs with male survivors. Porn addiction, promiscuity, lack of sexual interest, and fetishes are a few of the common sexual issues I have seen. Many of these sexual manifestations are a result of boundaries being crossed during sexual abuse.

Control is another avenue that survivors use to cope with their abuse. I am not referring to the kind of control that is prevalent in abusive relationships, but rather the kind of control that makes a person feel safe. When survivors were abused as children, they had no control over what happened to them. As adults they use control to protect themselves. Many survivors, Robert included, want to control the flow of the relationship. They carefully manipulate the dynamics, such as how close they allow you to get to them and what you think of them. Maybe they limit how often you see one another or when. They want to control how the relationship works in order to put themselves in a position where they perceive they cannot be harmed, physically, emotionally, financially or otherwise.

Other male survivors don't use any of these outlets and instead push people away. When you try to go deeper in a relationship, they pull back. When you reach inside to see what is there, they evaporate like vapor, never allowing you near enough to see their truly vulnerable side.

The suffering and aftermath of abuse does not discriminate. It touches men of all ages and all backgrounds. The male survivor's pain and how his abuse has impacted his life may be viewed unclearly or as "baggage." While this is not entirely accurate, it can be understood as an attitude of someone who may not know better, who may feel ill-equipped to engage with someone who has such a past or see men as having to fit a culturally prescribed suit of invulnerability. Numerous women find meaningful and lasting bonds with significant others who have experienced abuse and have undergone or are continuing the process of healing from the consequences of trauma.

Chapter 6

Should I Stay or Should I Go?

"STOP IT!" I screamed at Robert as he slammed on the brakes. Robert and I were both hysterical – me with fear and him with anger. All the trauma he had ever experienced was channeling through him at that moment. Our 3-year-old son Lawrence remained calm in the backseat of the car, analyzing the situation for a solution, which he usually does.

Moments before, a man had cut us off in traffic, but Robert's rage wasn't about that. It was about everyone who had ever slighted him. As he continued driving, he was becoming increasingly upset and angry. I could see the pain cutting through his eyes as he yelled at me not to tell him what do.

It was my birthday that day, and we had spent the day in Orange County with my family celebrating. Before we left that morning, Robert said how he hated Orange County because "the people down there are pretentious." The comment struck me at the time as off, but later, I saw that it had been a projection of his feelings and a premonition of what was to come. Throughout the day, his perceptions of the people of Orange County festered in his mind and built up. The other driver was merely the trigger for the explosion and venting of his pent up feelings.

I was more upset at him than I had ever been. I wasn't angry, but rather deeply saddened and disappointed. He had allowed himself to lose his temper in a dramatic fashion, with our son sitting in the back seat. Lawrence could have been seriously injured, possibly witness his father get arrested or at the very least experience some sort of trauma himself. All these possibilities ran through my head, making me more upset as the seconds ticked by.

Lawrence tried to help, exclaiming several times, "Go that way!" and pointing home. Here were Robert and I both pumped up on adrenaline ready to fire with a 3-year-old boy rationally trying to get us on track. But my brain kept reminding me of the fact that his safety was at risk. It was a thought loop I couldn't break out of, and it struck a nerve in my soul.

If there was any time that I was going to leave Robert, it was then. Frankly, if it weren't for Lawrence, I would've gotten out of that car and never looked back. I would've disconnected and disappeared completely, which is something I am good at when I want a person out of my life. The event affected me so deeply that it put me on the crossroads of having to decide whether to stay with my husband or leave for good.

There was a lot to think about on the ride home, and even more so when we arrived. He sat in the bedroom while I collapsed on to my father and cried in his lap for several hours. Over the next several days, Robert and I did not speak to one another except out of necessity, and that gave me the space I needed to sit in solitude and honestly decide what would be best for me and my family.

I thought about all the reasons to stay and leave, what life would be like without him, and if I was willing to accept that. The weight of this decision was a heavy burden that I carried around for the next several weeks. It was so heavy that I looked like I was physically carrying it. On one of those days, I was sitting in my office trying to get some work done when I drifted off into the memory of when we met.

I was living in California, he was living in Chicago, and we talked for several months online before meeting in person. The American Psychological Association conference was in Chicago that year, and I was planning to fly out, go to the conference, and meet Robert.

When I landed in Chicago, he met me at the airport to greet me, but I didn't let him pick me up. I possess a hypervigilance that has worsened over the years as a result of the work I do. I wasn't about to let a man I never met pick me up from the airport. Instead, I rented a car and went to my hotel. I thought it sweet of him to come and greet me anyway.

The following day Robert picked me up and we went on our first date. We drove all the way to Indiana to see Richard Speck's house. Speck was a mass murderer in Chicago who killed eight women in the '60s. Afterward, he took me to a pizza parlor for lunch. As I sat in that parlor, I knew, in the middle of a slice of pizza, that I was going to marry that man. The date may have been odd for most people, but my work has centered on a fascination of the extremes of human psychology. And I love pizza. Robert knew I would enjoy the outing because he had picked up on the kind of person I was – my likes and interests. He had paid attention to who I was.

Money and things like fancy restaurants, glitz and glamour mean nothing to me. That's all fun to look at and partake in from time to time, but they are superficial novelties. I am not interested in that. I want to get to know people on deeper planes – find out what drives them, discover their joys and fears.

Robert gave me something that no amount of money could purchase, the most valuable thing we possess – time. He also intuitively knew what carried weight in my soul. It was effortless, as if he was already programmed to know this without having to think about it. There are only a handful of times in my life that I have instantly connected with someone on this deeper plane. It convinced me that I would marry him. These memories swirled in my head for days, even appearing in my dreams. They were juxtaposed with the reality of the inventory of our marriage that I had to take.

After I had honestly analyzed our relationship, I made the decision to stay. I took an in-depth look at his behavior, how he treated Lawrence, and how he treated me. I came to realize I would much rather live with Robert's trauma and work through it with him than cut ties and start over.

The first question anyone should ask themselves when deciding whether to stay or go in a relationship is: Is this relationship abusive or does it have the potential to be abusive? For me that answer was an unequivocal "no." Robert would never abuse my son or me - not now, not ever.

The truth is that behavior like that Robert exhibited in Orange County had only been occurring since Lawrence was born. Robert always had a chip on his shoulder, wanting to be the biggest, toughest guy in the room, but after we had Lawrence it became bigger and more frantic. Everything and everyone became a perceived threat to our son, which manifested from the trauma Robert carried. This kind of reaction and behavior could be dealt with as Robert went further in his journey of processing his childhood trauma.

Robert is a phenomenal father to our son. He goes above and beyond to provide a one of a kind experience for him that no man could duplicate. No man can be the father that Robert is to Lawrence. He is always present in our son's life. On weekends they disappear for hours into the garage to tinker and build things. He teaches him, takes him to extracurricular activities, and provides Lawrence with a masculine presence that I cannot give him as his mother. I would never trust anyone else but Robert to raise our son.

Robert and I also have a connection that can't be duplicated. Despite our many differences we are very similar in our tastes and mindsets, especially when it comes to raising our son. Our roles as parents are symbiotic and intertwined; removing one of us from the dynamic would be detrimental to Lawrence.

I have never met another human being that I connect with like Robert; he is truly my best friend. Our relationship is completely open and honest; we have no secrets and share everything. I know there is absolutely nothing I cannot tell him. He understands me on a deep mental, emotional, and spiritual level.

A connection like the one we have is extremely rare in life – some people never find it – and I know that if I were to leave him I would never have a relationship like this again.

I thought about all that Robert does for us, the true expressions of his love, the intangibles that cannot be measured but make all the difference. Last summer I was speaking in Geneva at the United Nations on the topic of male trauma and how it relates to gang intervention – another issue I am passionate about. The U.N. summit was five days long at the beginning of July, which is also when the SCRIPT conference for male survivors takes place. I was to fly from Los Angeles to Geneva on Tuesday, return on a Sunday, and attend SCRIPT, which I set up and manage, top to bottom, the following Tuesday morning. If that weren't enough, my 4-year-old son and parents had to be driven from our house to downtown Los Angeles, a two-hour trip. Despite my desire to control and manage situations, I had to throw my hands up on this one. There was no way I could be in two places at once.

Robert handled everything from the big details of the conference to the minor details of Lawrence's clothes and even mine. When I arrived at the hotel in downtown Los

Angeles, Robert had my blue dress on a hanger in the closet. He had a checklist with everything that needed to get done. He had a plan for my family who were coming into town for the conference. He got Lawrence and my mother ready, and drove them to Los Angeles. Without his help, that SCRIPT conference would've been a nightmare for me, one of the few times I'll admit I could not have done that on my own.

But that is Robert: he goes the extra mile for our family without question. That is what counts, and in my eyes that is what love is. I choose to focus on the things I love about him, why I fell for him in the first place. That is 80% of our relationship. When I did that, the answer to stay became obvious to me.

After I made that decision, we needed to use some tools to make the relationship healthier and sustainable. Having been with Robert nearly 15 years, I know a few things about what makes him tick, and I know he has made significant progress dealing with his trauma through the years.

When I first met him he had not dealt with it at all. We were at ground zero, and he was fresh out of a 15-year marriage with a woman who was more or less another abuser so there was a lot to work through. We made great progress together, navigating the issues slowly, and then Lawrence was born. While the birth of Lawrence made certain areas of our life blossom, it unearthed the trauma that Robert had not dealt with and brought it front and center. This created a new challenge for us, and an opportunity to grow in a new way together that we still work through to this day.

The first thing I had to realize – and what all parents have to come to terms with – is that when my son was born, life no longer was all about me. Life changes forever the day we have children, and our own needs have to take a backseat to theirs.

When dealing with Robert's trauma and how it manifests, my first thought can't be *Well, this offends me* or *I don't like that*. I had to shift my focus onto what mattered – my son and the family unit. First, the question has to be framed as to "How does this affect my son?" and second, "How does this affect us as a family unit?" When I shift my focus and begin with these two questions, it allows me to deal with any problem that arises in an honest and productive way that is always keeping the welfare of my son in the foreground.

Putting myself second is necessary. When it comes time to address how Robert's issues affect me, I am able to view them from a different perspective. When addressing our relationship, I often come from the mindset that Robert can't function without me. I handle the finances and often make decisions for him. Before he met me he existed but was not living. His relationships were dysfunctional, like the one with his first wife. When he and I met, it became clear that we completed one another.

For our relationship to function, I had to learn to separate "the trauma" from the man. I can't change his trauma because it has nothing to do with me; it was present long before he ever met me, and manifestations of that trauma are not directed at me personally. I had to stop trying to change him and accept him for who he is – the good and the bad. I didn't cause his trauma, I can't cure it, and I can't control it; he needs to have his own experience and process with it.

All I can control is myself, my actions, and my reactions. Many of our arguments and fights were a result of minor disagreements that gained momentum by going tit for tat, eventually blowing up into screaming matches.

We argued over things like Facebook. He'd say, "All you do is post selfies of yourself," to which I would reply something along the lines of "it's not your Facebook." Clearly, this is a pointless argument. It only carries the potential to roll downhill into a much bigger snowball. But I realized that if I didn't engage in that type of exchange, there would be no blowup. So I started to choose to let the moment be, and let his meaningless comments roll by without engaging in them. In a day, week, or month will this matter? If I can answer "probably not" to that question, I walk away from arguments.

It is much more important for me to be happy than for me to be right. I choose to be happy over being right – even if I am right – and our relationship has improved dramatically because of it. You have to pick and choose your battles. Every couple has frivolous arguments. The trick is to not continue them into a realm that becomes personal and hurtful.

Adding positive, bonding experiences is another profound change in our relationship. I am not interested in simply avoiding negative experiences. I want to foster new, positive ones for us and Lawrence.

I always share with people that my dream is to have everyone I love living in the same house so that I never have to live without them. I want my family and friends around all the time. Although it is just a happy daydream I slide off into sometimes, I have made part of this a reality with Robert and Lawrence. We do everything together. We have a great social life visiting friends and family, taking day trips to Disneyland or the zoo. We actively enjoy spending time with one another. This helps ease the stress any of us feels in our lives because there is the common experience that we are in this together as one cohesive unit.

It's also important for me and Robert to have our own time to foster intimacy between us. A few times a month we have a date night where we go out to dinner or see a movie. Emotional and physical intimacy is difficult for him, and date nights can be stressful for him to plan, so I take the initiative with them. It helps us to decompress and grow closer with one another, though often times we can't wait to get home to our son.

I also use activity as a tool for distraction when I have to. If I know Robert is in one of his moods, I will suggest we all do something – Disneyland, movies, anything – that will get him outside of his head and focus on whatever it is we are doing.

Much of my success in choosing to stay and then maintaining and growing our relationship has been a result of changing my perception. I focus on the things I love about Robert – the reasons I fell in love with him and married him in the first place, and everything he does for us. When he acts out in erratic behavior, I recognize it as trauma, and allow him the space he needs to express that. I try to stay on my side of the street and keep control over my words and actions – I can't control him. I have come to understand that he sees the world through different eyes than I do, and that has fostered new compassion and growth in me.

Chapter 7

Should You Stay or
Should You Go?

Loren M. Hill, Ph.D.

The Chicago School of Professional Psychology
Los Angeles, Ca.

The question of "Should I stay or should I go?" has run through the minds of most spouses/partners of male survivors. It can be a deep conflict, like a tug of war in your mind that results in a stalemate, which can be frustrating to a spouse desperately looking for an answer. Kids, finances, extended family – where do I even start? How do I even go about leaving? Or even more puzzling: how do I go about staying? We navigate this process one step at a time, thinking through each question honestly and thoroughly, using tools proven to give us better insight to our relationship and ourselves.

Whatever you choose, staying or leaving, you want to feel confident that you have made the best possible choice for you and your family. By exploring the options, you have, based on your unique situation, you give yourself the best opportunity to be happy and healthy.

Abuse can be physical, verbal, emotional, or even financial. Physical abuse includes striking, slapping, punching, or kicking your partner and presents the most imminent threat to your safety. Verbal and emotional abuse like name calling, derogatory or demeaning language, and threats can be just as psychologically damaging (or more so) than physical abuse and should not be brushed off.

Financial abuse occurs when one partner restricts money from the other partner. Usually in a relationship one party is better at handling the finances and takes on that responsibility – that is not abuse. A financially abusive relationship is a relationship that is a one-way street, where one of the parties has no say in financial matters. When one partner controls the money in a way that involves fear, control, coercion or threats, it is considered financial abuse. If someone is scared to spend money because they will be hit, verbally abused or berated, they are experiencing financial abuse. If they "must" turn over their paycheck and are given an "allowance" with no input on decision-making, that is abusive.

The essence of the abusive relationship is that it is not a partnership. There is one person who dominates and controls the dynamic of the relationship through fear and coercion. Coercion means control or dominance over someone else through the use of physical, emotional, or sexual abuse.

There are very few conversations in an abusive relationship. They are one-sided lectures where the abuser berates the other person. A conversation over money could look like the abuser calling their partner names or telling them how stupid they are for paying the rent with money they were saving to buy a car.

In a non-abusive relationship, the conversations are amicable discussions where two partners work together to achieve a common goal. That same conversation about money will be constructive, even in times of conflict. *We are on a budget because we need to save for a new car* is an example of the same conversation over money, spoken with a much more constructive perspective.

I have worked with people whose entire experience in a relationship has been abuse. They say things such as *Nothing you're describing is outside of the norm for our relationship.*

We can't define things as normal or not normal, because abuse may be the norm for that relationship. Instead, we have to look at the dynamics of the relationship from the perspective of healthy vs. not healthy.

Using the example of finances, since it is a topic that every couple deals with and can often produce heated discussions, a healthy conversation is a shared, two-way dialogue of why we can or can't afford something. We don't use these types of routine conversations with our spouse as battlefields to unload the stress we picked up throughout our day.

An unhealthy conversation results in one party ignoring the other, making them feel inferior, or less intelligent, and can escalate into screaming, threats, intimidation, and violence. Deciding whether to stay or go could be the biggest question you face in your life. It is important that you think through everything thoroughly and without outside distractions.

People tend to lose themselves in their relationships, especially if they have been with that person for a significant part of their life. The lives of two people become so intertwined that they may not know who they are as individuals. Many times people sacrifice their needs for the greater good of the relationship. When faced with the possibility of being without that other person, it is necessary that you explore yourself. Your needs now may be much different from those you had when you met your partner. You have undoubtedly changed since that time and have become a different person. It is essential to your wellbeing to explore that.

There are many tools you can use to help you explore yourself and the dynamic of your relationship. Those tools will be crucial in coming to a solid decision of what your best option is. I have found in my clinical work, as well as my personal life, that nothing beats putting pen to paper or fingers to keyboard. Things become much clearer to us when we write them down as opposed to just thinking them through in our heads. They become permanent and real, and we can watch ourselves work through problems in a tangible way.

A great place to start is by creating a pros/cons list, but do it twice from different perspectives. The first list will be: *Why should I stay?* vs. *Why should I go?* This list will contain things like: I love my kids, my house, and my current lifestyle or I don't like my current lifestyle. This is more pertinent to the specific life situation you are in and will take into account the many outside factors that will influence your choice. The second list is much more personal and should be titled: *Why I am with him?* vs. *Why I shouldn't be with him?*, and will be specific to the relationship between you and your partner. On this list you will write things like I love John or John is abusive to me in this way: emotional, physical, sexual, or financial.

Another great tool is writing down what your life may be like if you stay vs. what it might be like if you leave. You'll want to ask yourself: *If I leave, where will I go? Who will I tell? Where will I work?*

Many times people leave relationships abruptly – sometimes out of necessity, as in the case of abusive relationships, without thinking about the other serious life decisions that have to be made when life is uprooted and drastically changed. Practical logistics need to be worked out beforehand, such as putting the kids in a new school and securing first and last month's rent for an apartment. The details need to be worked out beforehand to make transitioning easier on you and the kids. The daily activities and routine of all involved may change dramatically, and you should be prepared for that.

However, if you are in an abusive relationship, do not write anything down. He may find what you have written, which could result in physical harm to you or your kids. Your first priority is staying safe. Instead, seek help immediately from a domestic violence hotline. Counselors will guide you on a safe exit strategy, and provide resources you and your children will need upon leaving the relationship.

Finally, if you need to talk to someone, talk to someone outside of the relationship who has is impartial and not biased toward the outcome of your relationship. It is not wise to bounce these ideas off friends and family members. Although they mean well, they will have an emotional attachment to the situation one way or another, and their advice may be clouded by their emotions. It is best to talk to a therapist or similar third party, not necessarily a couples counselor, but an individual therapist, as this decision is specific to you. If you wish to try couples counseling first, that could be beneficial. It may give you a clearer picture of the situation and point you more confidently in the direction of staying or going.

It is important to keep in mind that this is a solitary process. It is in your best interest to think it through without any outside interference – positive or negative. Be mindful about discussing your exploration of staying or leaving with your partner. You may tell him you want to leave, expecting him to beg you to stay. Instead he tells you to pack your bags and leave. In reality he is responding from a place of fear, seeking to isolate, and not wanting to deal with his own issues.

Throughout the decision-making process it is necessary to keep the healthy dialogue flowing and to foster it as much as possible. Countless women have said to me, *This is still the guy I love. We just stopped talking.*

There will not be a greater factor in your decision than your children. Their well-being is paramount, and all of your decisions need to be made with this in mind. Many people say you have to stay for the kids, and too often couples stay in toxic relationships for what they perceive is the best interest of the children. This is not accurate. If every sign is pointing you to leave, and the only thing holding you back is the children, it might be best to go. Staying for the kids will create a long-term toxic relationship, which will be detrimental to all involved, including the kids. If it is feasible, you can always co-parent.

Children mimic the behavior they grow up around, and act out with future partners, the behaviors learned from their parents. If a house is full of discord, then that is what they will learn. All things being equal, maintaining the nuclear family is a good idea, but if the household is toxic and unhealthy, this will be the learned behavior the children pick up on, and the repercussions could last a lifetime.

Children do not get enough credit for their intelligence. They take in the world on a context basis rather than content. This means that they pick up on non-verbal cues very well and can tell when words don't match actions. They notice the inconsistency of people's actions. Kids are like little satellite dishes taking in all of the information around them. They pick up on everything.

The point is that you have to honestly assess the kind of relationship the kids are learning. You are modeling behavior for them every day, positive and negative. So while the children should not be the sole motivator for staying, they can also be a great motivator to stay as you will get to show them a healthy relationship where you and your husband/partner are working through problems and establishing healthy boundaries.

If you make the decision to leave, you will still get the opportunity to show your children healthy interactions through the way you and your ex co-parent. Additionally, demonstrating how to stand up for yourself in an abusive situation is an invaluable lesson.

A conversation with your husband/partner on the logistics of co-parenting will make the transition easier on the kids, as well as on both of you. Matters like where they will live and where they will go to school are necessary to work through together, hopefully in an amicable way. If a constructive conversation is not possible, you can file papers in Family Court and let a judge decide physical/legal custody and give binding orders on the logistics.

If you get a divorce/separate, you can't skirt around the court issue. The children will be a part of the legal proceedings, but should be protected from the discussions of what is happening. Custody will be a part of that, as well. When possible you and your partner should make every effort to resolve custody issues between the two of you. Remember the primary goal of the court is determining what is in the best interest of the children and not what is most convenient for the parents.

Rules of engagement are crucial to co-parenting in a healthy, constructive way. Ask your ex what he expects from you as a parent and tell him what you expect, as well. Make your intentions clear and set firm boundaries to avoid disputes – legal or otherwise – down the road.

Have an agreement that both of you will be fully present in the children's lives. They want to see both of their parents at their activities such as baseball games and dance recitals. This agreement includes the fun and not-so-fun stuff, meaning you will both have to discipline the children, as well. There shouldn't be the "when I go to mom's/dad's house, he/she lets me do what I want." Consistency and continuity need to be maintained in the way you discipline each of your children.

Sometimes circumstances are such that it is nearly impossible to co-parent with your ex. In situations like this, the priority should always be protecting the children. The easiest way to protect your children is through the legally through the court system. If your ex is violent or you fear he has the potential be abusive, get a restraining order! Restraining orders will cover your home, work, the children's school, and any other places you list.

Court-monitored visits are another useful tool. You can arrange with the court that your ex must be monitored when he is with the children.

The most important thing is to remember that the children are off-limits in disputes between you and your ex. Do not recruit them on your side or project onto them your negative feelings about your ex. Don't talk in a derogatory manner about your ex to your children, either. All of this creates significant confusion in the child's life and trauma that your child will have to process later as an adult. Healthy boundaries between you, your ex, and the children are keys to co-parenting; healthy outlets (like therapy) will help you maintain those boundaries.

Healthy outlets for everyone, especially the kids, may make leaving a lot easier. Encourage healthy emotional responses for everyone. If your child feels like crying, let them cry. Giving them their space and allowing them to process emotions in a way they see fit, helps them work through the situation. Children are far more resilient than we think.

Be open to talking with your children, and be honest about the situation. They can pick up on what is going on anyway. Engaging them in age appropriate conversations about what is going on with mom and dad is beneficial to their growth and well-being.

A healthy plan to remain, and tools that will help foster a healthy relationship, is paired with the decision to stay. First, ask your spouse if he wants you to stay. This may seem obvious but is often an afterthought. The two of you need to work as a team. It will be worth knowing that he desires your presence in the relationship and is on the same page about taking the steps necessary to create a healthy relationship. Decide what you are able to accept, and come to an understanding of what is and isn't acceptable as you move through this journey with him.

Also let him know why you want to stay with him. When thinking of the reasons why you are staying, think of the reasons you fell in love with him in the first place. It is also healthy and beneficial to revisit these memories from time to time. It helps keep the relationship in perspective. As you remind yourself of those reasons, remind him of them too. Tell him why you love him and why you want to stay with him. Remember that he views the world through different lenses than you do, and much of that world view is based on the trauma he suffered as a child.

The trauma makes a male survivor withdrawn and can make you feel inadequate, as if you are failing. As you try to pull information from him through the course of your daily interactions, if he withdraws and retreats, it is helpful to understand that it has nothing to do with you. It is not a personal attack on you. A male survivor hasn't been able to open up with anyone. He does not have the skills to effectively verbalize how he is feeling.

You have made the decision to stay, and he has given his commitment to the process. He will need to find a way to communicate his feelings, disclose his past abuse, and seek treatment. This can be done through couples counseling, individual therapy, or support groups. He has to have his own way of healing and be open to that process. As the spouse, all you can do is support that process. It does not happen overnight, and it is very much a three steps forward, two steps back, kind of process.

Every healthy relationship uses a variety of tools to increase intimacy, defuse stress, and strengthen the bonds formed between two people. For the spouse/partner who is in a relationship with a male survivor, these same tools are more important than in your average relationship.

Troubles with intimacy, both emotional and physical, are hallmark problems in relationships with male survivors. Creating a space for the intimacy to grow is a powerful tool to use in your relationship. Intimacy is physical, emotional, and mental and doesn't always have to culminate in intercourse. When trying to foster sexual intimacy, there is no need to force it. Intimacy will look different for every couple. The point is that you are spending positive time with one another.

Sexual intimacy can be difficult for male survivors, and as a spouse/partner, remember it is not about you. Some days he will be triggered more than other days. There should be a mutual code of understanding that it is not about a lack of attraction to you, but rather the innate anxiety that sexual intimacy can produce in male survivors. You can still have positive growth in physical intimacy with cuddling, spooning, or just an intimate conversation. All of these are beneficial in the bigger picture of creating physical intimacy with your partner.

Rejection is a common feeling for spouses/partners of male survivors. There is no sugar-coating it – it feels terrible. You think you are the problem. You simply cannot fix it. It has nothing to do with you. Your husband/partner might try to make it about you, *You're not attracted to me. You don't do the things you used to.* Then you try and do those things, and it still doesn't work. I have to emphasize this point – it is not about you, your appearance, performance, or anything else.

Have a space in your calendar devoted to just the two of you, like a date night. You both get to decide what you do on that night. If the house is distracting, leave. The outing does not have to be extravagant or lavish. If all you can budget is McDonald's, go eat at McDonald's, but go inside the restaurant, sit down, and eat together. All that matters is that you are spending time alone enjoying each other's company. It should be sacred time.

There also needs to be a designated night of the week where you spend time together as a family unit. This could be a game night, movie night, or bowling night. The goal is to build intimacy with one another as a family – learn to talk with each other on a deeper level, meaning turn off the cell phones and video games and put away the electronic devices. Have dinner together as a family where you all talk about your day. It seems basic, but in the digital age, we seem to have lost this connection with our family members through distractions like smart phones.

Also set aside time to talk about your relationship with your partner. Each week, have an inventory process with each other. It doesn't have to be long, just an hour a week will do. Discuss things like what is and isn't working in the relationship or do a weekly budget review, if financials are a communal matter of dispute. How to do this weekly inventory process will be a matter of trial and error. You may find one way works, while another doesn't. The only way to find out is to make an effort and try different styles until one sticks. The style of a set weekly schedule is beneficial because it ensures that you both will sit down and talk.

When a male survivor gets angry, it is hard for them to verbalize what they are feeling. They can seem to go blind with rage, unable to explain what is going on inside them. Talking this over during a weekly inventory is extremely beneficial because it removes both of you from the emotion of the moment. You can go back to the situation during the inventory and review it with a calmer mind and different perspective. If they get angry during the inventory process, it is best to shut it down and walk away. They will be unable to hear you in a meaningful way and the conversation can degrade into an argument quickly. Many times, the spouse unintentionally pulls the triggers that set off the male survivor. You need to have the insight to walk away and come back to it later when things have cooled off. It is not about you.

How you interact with one another is the biggest adjustment the two of you will have to make. If the way you used to interact wasn't working and created a lot of stress within the relationship, you need to establish new rules of engagement.

As a spouse/partner you have to be sensitive to how far you can push your spouse/partner in talking about their abuse and discussing his feelings. It is like peeling an onion back layer by layer. It will occur over time, but forcing your spouse to talk about something he is uncomfortable with, is not beneficial to either one of you, and is actually counterproductive, as he may have the tendency to retreat further into his shell.

There is also a time and place to address conflicts with your spouse. Some spouses feel they are being attacked when they confronted with conflict in public. Others don't want to engage in front of the kids. You have to find the proper time to deal with conflict. The weekly inventory meeting can work, but don't let this become a routine complaint session, or it will lose its value. The weekly meeting is for processing issues, moving forward, and growing from them. Emotions often influence us to act in the moment. We feel like we need to say something right away, but that is not always true, and in fact usually is not. Sometimes it's beneficial to just sit with the moment and let it pass. Let the moment just be a moment. It is not realistic to disengage when you are upset, but you can take steps to mitigate the damage.

A great tool to use is the three questions: *Does it need to be said? Does it need to be said by me? Does it need to be said by me right now?* This simple tool is helpful in avoiding unnecessary fights and can change the entire dynamic of your relationship.

Come to an agreement on shared rules of engagement, a shared code. Don't dehumanize one another through name-calling or profanity, belittling or disrespecting. Always engage each other in a humanizing way that shows respect for one another. This shared code is not one that is established at the beginning of the relationship and then forgotten about. It has to be constant. As the spouse/partner, you should maintain your side of the rules of engagement and keep those boundaries firm. Statements such as *Please do not speak to me like that. I will not tolerate abusive language,* are healthy ways to maintain that shared code. If he steps over the line, the best thing to do is disengage and walk away. Maintaining the rules of engagement – your shared code –has to fall on you, the spouse/partner. When a male survivor is triggered and enters that state of anger, everything else is blocked out.

Most of the tools we covered do not require major changes in your lifestyle, but rather are minor tweaks that are simple in nature and easy to implement, but have profound results in relationships. They will also empower you as a spouse/partner to set and enforce boundaries. With these tools you can take an active approach to healing your relationship and planting it in healthier ground, giving it the conditions you both need to grow.

Chapter 8

Anger is the Engine

Anger is the engine that drives many of the outbursts, isolation, and distancing I have described. It is the seed from which all other issues grow.

I had a seething anger against Robert's abusers. Most of it I have worked through, and some of it I have not. But for years I carried anger at the people who damaged my husband, and that affected him, our son, and me.

The only person I didn't have anger towards was his first wife. It might come off of as strange because of the trauma she put him through, but she was just as unhealthy as he was. She had bipolar disorder, and he was a male survivor whose trauma had not yet begun to surface. They were two unhealthy people who had found each other and were living out an unhealthy relationship. She was not equipped with tools to deal with Robert's trauma. Their relationship did not stand a chance at being successful and healthy.

I was the child of parents who were divorced and remarried. Growing up, I had the examples of my mother working together with her ex-husband to raise my brothers. My parents never used their kids as pawns, pitting the kids against the other parent. They were good role models on co-parenting.

I never had much anger towards Sammy. He abused Robert at the age of 12. For a child to do that, he clearly had some deep-seated issues. He probably was a victim of abuse and was simply acting out what he knew.

My source of deep, red-hot anger was directed at the adults who abused Robert because they could not control themselves. Their actions directly led to Robert's lifelong issues, ones that I have to deal with on a daily basis. Most of that anger was directed at Robert's aunt. It has been a difficult journey navigating that anger because the aunt's abuse is the source of all of Robert's issues surrounding women that really affect my life. The trauma of the abuse is acted out in all aspects of a survivor's life.

Another deep source of my anger, which in all likelihood you share as a spouse, was my husband. The origins of this anger come from the fact that Robert knew he had issues and he knew they were deeply rooted in trauma. However, he painted a picture of holding it together. In all fairness, his holding back was not deliberate. Someone isn't going to come out and tell you he is a male survivor during the courting process. That just isn't how it works. He didn't know the ripple effect his trauma would have on every aspect of our lives, and he still doesn't realize it like I do. I have to live with the consequences of his trauma, and I live on the receiving end.

While a male survivor can weave an appearance of normalcy into their lives, trauma is a thread running through it, which if pulled, will unravel them. For years I thought I was crazy. I thought it was all in my head. Once the truth comes to light, anger is one of the most appropriate feelings I can think of. It was in my case.

The thread that runs through survivors' lives is the trauma. When the thread of trauma is pulled, intentionally or not, the male survivor acts out in behaviors such as anger, "hiding under the covers," or passive aggression. That thread is the source of great instability and unpredictability. In my relationship, as in many relationships of male survivors, the cycle looks like this: There is a period of normality, where they are engaging, open, and communicative. Eventually you do something that they perceive as critical or insensitive. Maybe you are not listening or you tell them you want some space, you are worn out. This boundary setting is perceived as a slight that starts a phase of passive aggressive behavior by the survivor. This can last for weeks. Eventually this leads to the survivor blowing up in a fit of anger. *You never listen to me! You don't care about me!* or some variation of these feelings. Finally, after they cool down, everything goes back to normal and the cycle resets. In my relationship with Robert, the closer he felt to me over the years, the nastier he would be to me during those blow up stages. As a spouse, this cycle can be miserable to live in. It is unstable and unpredictable at times and becomes a well of resentment and anger.

There are periods of anger and walking on eggshells that seem like they will never end. As a spouse, I wonder whether he wants me around or not.

When he is in one of these periods, there is nothing I can say that is right. Every comment becomes a contested point. There must be something behind it - a hidden agenda or manipulation. You ask a question, one they happen to not have an answer for, and they become angry and frustrated, turning everything back onto you – *You're always nagging me! Quit badgering me!* It wears you out, especially when you have no idea where it is coming from. It is as random and unpredictable as the weather, and when the hurricane comes, there is nothing we can do but board up the windows and wait it out.

This cycle is only about 20% of our relationship. The rest of the time we have a great relationship. But during that fraction of instability, he rarely resembles the man I know. He becomes irritable and lashes out frequently or sulks and is avoidant.

As a spouse, that anger builds up over the years. It has to be released, or it will explode. It can be a lonely journey sometimes since you are not able to express how you feel. You can't talk to your spouse because you don't want to set him off in the heat of the moment. It is difficult to talk to family and friends because you fear they may judge you or won't understand. Keeping all of these feelings inside can bring us to a lonely and dark place within ourselves. It did for me.

When Lawrence was 6 months old, all of my anger exploded at once. Twelve long years of bottled emotions erupted in a cataclysmic fashion. My vision went red. I was screaming so much that my vocal chords ached and spit was flying from my mouth. The odd thing is I can't even remember why. My brain blocked out the memory. But that was when I hit the bedrock of my anger. From there I realized I could not have an outburst like that again. I had to change. It wasn't on him to control this. It was up to me. This anger did not serve me. My anger could not allow me to go back into the past and change what happened to my husband. It wouldn't motivate him to change or deal with his issues. It was an empty emotion and poison to my soul.

Before I had an understanding of my husband, his abuse, and how it manifests, I was completely blindsided by his mood swings. I had no understanding that they stemmed from the abuse he experienced, and how abuse ruins a survivor's sense of self. This response to trauma became the fundamental fact behind the mood swings my husband goes through.

My husband's abuse took place over the course of several years. Many behaviors and warped perceptions become ingrained in a person after being abused over any significant amount of time. The abuser has no regard for the victim's well-being. Emotional and physical control is what is being sought. The abuser manipulates the victim to believe that they have no control. As a result, they essentially lose their sense of self.

Lack of trust is a major residual effect of the abuse. It can stay with a survivor for the rest of his life. What is crucial, and may be very beneficial for you to understand, is that it is not just you he is scared to be vulnerable with – it is everyone. Men in our society are already trained not to show a wide range of emotions. They are told by society that they can only show two emotions – happiness and anger. This message constricts survivors tighter than other men.

A male survivor hasn't been allowed to express the full range of emotions. Society has told him he is not allowed, and his abuser told him that his emotions were irrelevant. That kind of trauma dies hard. Often times I describe my husband as having one speed. He only knows how to go 100 miles per hour. I've found that to be common with many men, not just survivors. Becoming vulnerable and allowing oneself to express a full range of emotions is counterintuitive to most men and more so with the male survivor. It is important to recognize that male survivors have the full range of emotions as everyone does. But survivors have more difficulty than non-survivors bringing those emotions to the surface and expressing them.

Anger toward the abuser, and to some degree themselves, creates a cycle of social dysfunction and isolation. The survivor is scared to get too close to anyone. They won't allow themselves the vulnerability it takes to develop deep intimacy with another human being. Isolation becomes their defense mechanism. It keeps others from controlling them. Any question or comment on your part can be perceived as an indictment or a way to control them.

There is always going to be some level of confrontation in any relationship. Confronting your husband about little things, like leaving the seat up or letting the hot water run, to major issues like finances are universal issues couples deal with. A person who has not suffered abuse is theoretically able to express their emotions in a thoughtful way when confronted. Not so with the male survivor. They have difficulty expressing their feelings. Instead, they project them onto their spouse and then retreat into whatever it is that protects them from emotion – usually anger or isolation.

What spouses have to remember is that this problem was around long before we were. Our husbands have been dealing with these issues their entire lives. I certainly cannot come along now – 30 years after the fact – and change him. I cannot make him feel emotions, and I cannot heal his trauma. When I came to that realization, I could see everything in full color again. I could breathe again. I didn't have to carry his burden on my shoulders anymore. I freed myself by identifying the fact that I cannot change him. I don't remember the exact moment, but I do remember it happened during one our fights. I ran to the bathroom and just sat there on the toilet contemplating everything. That's when it came to me – he is not going to change. Either I learn to love what I have, even the broken part, or this is going to end in a very volatile way. From there I was free from the burden I put on myself. I could embrace the broken, forgive the broken, and love all of who he is.

While I was thinking, it occurred to me that there was a breakdown in our communication when we engaged each other from different points of view. Routine conversations like minor financial decisions or where to go for dinner, turned into fights that would carry on for days. I took a step back from the situation and thought back on those encounters, paying special attention to my part in the conflict.

Almost every conversation went like this: An event or situation would arise that bothered me. I would confront Robert about it, and he would respond. Then I would fire back a response – then he – then I – so on and so forth. There was no break in the action. It was a coil of dialogue that wound more tensely as each of us became angrier. Once I identified this pattern, I implemented changes to it. Rather than immediately responding to him – firing back a quick-witted response as soon as one came to mind – I paused. I allowed the conversation to breathe. I would hear him out, allow him to get his point across, and leave it at that. This didn't do anything to change him or his response. I gave up trying to change him. However, it completely changed how I responded to conflict. I slowed down the flow of dialogue, and kept my composure and peace. After I started doing this, explosive anger on my end became rare.

Remember, a male survivor's perspective tends to come from a place of abuse. The subconscious perception of a possible threat activates, and the brain responds according to that perceived threat. Therefore, male survivors can respond in a way that will keep you at a distance. They don't want to deal with emotions, and they feel threatened. Their response will reflect a subconscious desire to push you away, and will manifest as cutting you off or talking over you. This is when I walk away. The conversation will only deteriorate from here, and we will end up in yet another fight.

I suggest you let the conflict sit and let him digest what you said to him. By creating a break in the tension and action, it gives him a moment to reflect and take in the full significance of what you said. Let him come back on his own time. That is crucial. It has to be on his time. He cannot feel like he is being put into a corner or controlled. The response to a perceived threat will most likely be the same. It probably won't be instant either, at least it hasn't been in my experience. They need time to feel the emotion, digest it, and formulate a thoughtful response to what was said. As a spouse, I understand how difficult this is for you.

There are times where I don't get the consoling or loving reciprocation I want right away. Slowing down interactions, and stepping away from them when necessary, has significantly improved our communication by creating a less tense environment.

Lawrence was a year old when Robert was diagnosed with thyroid cancer. At one point, it was so bad he had to be quarantined for treatment. In all honesty, this saved our marriage. I was ready to leave, but I couldn't do that to him. The cancer forced me to take a look within myself, and get rid of the anger that was holding me back.

So I had to learn not to be angry, which is easier said than done. But I had to do it, with the same necessity as I have to eat and drink water. Anger is poison to the soul, and I was only getting sicker. I also did not want my son to see me get angry. I especially never wanted him to witness the kind of blow up I had with Robert a few months prior.

I'm not a naturally angry person. I am a person of love and light. I like making people happy, and at my core I see love in the world. But I was starting to lose that. I was becoming unrecognizable to myself, and instead, was turning into a product of the people who abused Robert. I could never let them have that. Life is too short to harbor anger like that. That fact alone is enough motivation. If I want a better future and to be free, I need to forgive and let go.

The first step was identification. I began paying attention to my mind, noticing when those feelings of anger and resentment bubbled up. For so many years, I was at the mercy of my feelings. They would come and go as they please. Before I was aware of them, they had a grip on me. But now I would constantly check in with myself to see what I was feeling and thinking. I could see the anger start to form when Robert would say something that bothered me, or acted out in a way that felt inappropriate to me. By practicing this enough, I started to catch the anger earlier and earlier, closer to the incident that precipitated it. By doing so, I could stop myself before I went down the rabbit hole of rage.

After I became acquainted with the way my mind was working, I tried to reshape my thoughts and view Robert through a lens of love and care. I had to focus on coming from a place of compassion, which I was thrust into when he was diagnosed with cancer. The mind is malleable and we can change the way we think. For me, simply being aware of the feelings that were coming up, and reminding myself that love and compassion was my code, changed everything.

Around this time, I started talking about my problems with people. That was something I never did before. For our entire relationship, I thought I was crazy. I thought the primary problem was me. When I considered leaving Robert, I thought that it made me a bad person and bad wife. I began talking to my mom and dad about my and Robert's relationship. I began to use situations from our marriage as examples in class, just not saying they were Robert and me. Then I started writing this book.

The more I talked about it with others, the more I realized I wasn't crazy. Other people validated my experience and encouraged me by telling me I was doing the best I could. I was not pushing buttons or pulling triggers. Those buttons and triggers were present in Robert before he met me, and I cannot fix that. I decided I wasn't going to be angry with myself for something I did not cause, cannot control, or cure. His trauma, and its manifestations in our lives, had nothing to do with me. This was one of the most empowering realizations of my life, and the empowerment came when I started talking about it.

When his mother would call me asking how Robert was doing, which she frequently did, I told her she should call him herself. I'm not a caretaker or his mother, and I have no power over him or how he reacts to situations.

I also prayed. A lot. I had to get back to my spiritual roots and trust in God. I never prayed much until I was faced with this adversity. I just wanted my anger, and the feelings it spawned, to go away. I did not want to live in this misery anymore. I asked God to "make me light" again. Once I had the realization that I was going to be my own person of love and light again, I asked God to make it so. I found strength and comfort in this spiritual action, and it propelled me through the darkest and loneliest times in our marriage.

Once I had that awakening, which I hope you find as well, I had to maintain the space that was created. On a daily basis, I had to get in tune with my newfound awakening.

Gratitude is a simple way to do this. Instead of focusing on what our relationship lacked or what I felt I was not getting, I began to take inventory, and put more stock into what I have. I stopped chasing some unrealistic fairy tale fantasy of what a perfect marriage or a perfect husband is supposed to look like. Today, I stay in reality and realize what I have.

Since showing emotion can be difficult for Robert, I have to watch what he does to understand and know that he cares about me. I try to remember the old cliché: actions speak louder than words. You may get very few words from your husband, so train your eye to watch what he does. That is what counts. For a week before the second annual SCRIPT conference, Robert was running around like a mad man with a purpose, helping to get everything ready. He ironed tablecloths, went to Home Depot at midnight to buy me a dolly, made sure I had all my materials ready and organized.

People have a tendency to sit in misery because it is comfortable. They stay in bad marriages, work jobs they hate, and remain in toxic relationships because it is familiar to them. However, they aren't present in their lives. They "check out" through outlets such as extra-marital affairs, drugs and alcohol, or any other combination of distractions that will achieve the goal of getting their mind off of the negativity they have chosen to sit in.

This isn't the case with Robert. I can tell he is happy and present with his life. Although he has difficulty verbally expressing these emotions, he shows it by the countless hours he joyfully spends with Lawrence; he is present and enjoys when we do things together as a family. When we are getting ready to go on a vacation, I am excited for an entire week prior. I eagerly plan whole itineraries, but Robert remains stoic. "Aren't you excited!?" I'll say to him. "Yes. I'm looking forward to it," he says with his poker face. When we get to the destination, he is engaged and interested in what we are doing and contributes to the good time we have as a family. Robert is simply not as emotionally extroverted as I am. If I were not paying attention, I would miss the clues he leaves me.

Part of picking up these clues is training my intuition to look for them. I had to first identify that he was not emotionally extroverted and accept that. If I come to him with excitement over plans we have, expecting to get an excited response in return, I am fishing for a reaction I probably won't receive. That isn't his fault; he is who he is. I am bringing my expectations of his reactions to the table. That isn't fair to him. Once I identified this, I could accept him for who he is and taper my expectations of who he should be and how he should act. Meanwhile, my intuition is telling me to look for different signs of how he shows me he cares. This was the beginning of a deeper level of communication and understanding with Robert.

However, it is still a rollercoaster. We will have several weeks in which everything is clicking together followed by a week of disorganized turmoil where he is triggered, angry, isolating and "hiding under the bed." I'll think, "Am I crazy? Weren't the last few weeks so smooth? Am I imagining things? No, Deb, you're not crazy, and the way he is acting has nothing to do with you."

Those periods of time where everything seems to fall in place effortlessly are wonderful. I desire to prolong them. I travel frequently for work, mostly to prisons throughout California and across the country at least once a month. I recharge my emotional batteries on these trips. By creating space, I maintain my internal equilibrium. I am able to extend the "normal" periods of our relationship. I find these trips create balance in my life and allow me to catch my breath when I feel things getting tight.

Not everyone travels for work or has the means to travel on a regular basis. But all of us have the means to create healthy space. When I wasn't traveling for work, I reached out to my support network. I used the same tool that gave me my awakening in the first place – reaching out and talking to others. It fills in the gaps and makes me feel whole. I also get to unload a lot of baggage that I would otherwise be carrying around inside. Talking to the people in my support network is also invaluable. When I need to discuss a situation that I think Robert's issues will get in the way of, I go to my support network. I tell him later on – we have no secrets – but in the moment, it is not always productive to take every issue to him. Sometimes I need to go to other people for problem-solving first.

I also have other outlets like hobbies I use to maintain my serenity. I love art and being creative. I'll draw with Lawrence or bejewel a cell phone case. It puts my mind somewhere else and gives me joy and peace.

I've gotten into fitness and boxing recently. For two hours, I can put my mind on pause, and the only thing I need to focus on is punching the bag. I don't think about anything else. It puts my mind into a meditative state, and I come out feeling rejuvenated and calm.

Finally, I try to help others whenever I can. As a psychologist, I'm fortunate enough to have the opportunity to help others all day long. But even when I'm not at work, I call friends or family and ask how they are doing. Then I just sit back and listen. Being of service to others – by doing or listening – gets me out of my own head. For those few minutes or hours when I listen to someone else, or help talk them through a problem, I am not thinking about myself.

For you, I encourage you to look at the actions of your spouse, and not judge based their words alone. Keep the focus on you, your behavior, and finding ways to improve the communication. Sometimes this means stepping away for some time. Allow a cool down period. Build a support network because you cannot take all of this on by yourself.

Hopefully, this chapter has given you a clearer picture of your spouse, what causes him to act the way he does, and your own reactions. We have only begun to tap into our understanding, and our own individual journeys will reveal more to you. My wish is that you have the necessary tools to navigate the rough times and maximize the joyful ones.

Chapter 9

SCRIPT – Summit on Community Resilience, Intervention, Prevention, and Training

Part One

Nikeisha Brooks, M.A.
The Chicago School of Professional Psychology
Psy.D. Student

Associate Director of Coordination
SCRIPT Conference

Growing up in the inner city I was surrounded by male survivors. Survivors of poverty, neglect, abuse, addiction, gang violence, police brutality, and incarceration. I recognized at an early age that there are significant differences in the experiences of males born and raised in the inner city compared to females. As I got older I began to understand many of the additional daily life stressors that men in my community had to endure, and the significant impact these stressors had on their family relationships, social interactions, and occupational performance.

I can personally relate to the negative impact on family relationships as I was raised by a single mother. My father was a part of my life from birth until age 6 and then he wasn't. I always resided with my mother, but prior to his departure, my father was a fairly constant figure in my life. Some of my earliest memories are of riding with him on his Harley with the stench of his cigar in my nostrils and thinking, "I have the coolest dad in the world!" Little did I know, he and I would one day be strangers. My father and I reconnected when I was 25. At the time, I didn't see the point, however, my family, and surprisingly my mother, insisted that I needed to see him face to face as though I was owed an explanation.

I wouldn't get that explanation for another five years or so. Spending time with him allowed me the opportunity to hear his story, which consisted of neglect, physical abuse, gang violence, and drugs. I began to understand generational patterns of dysfunction, and how his lack of a positive father figure in his life prevented him from learning and understanding what being a father means and how to be one. It was only after I understood his experience that I could accept him for who he was and have no expectations of him. Although he is not the typical father, he has made consistent efforts over the past 10 years to remain a part of my life – not so much as a parent, but as a friend, and that works for us. When I was first presented with the opportunity to work with SCRIPT, I had no idea where my motivation to agree came from, however, everything in me was telling me that the conference would be a significant part of my journey.

My role on the SCRIPT team is associate conference director with my main responsibilities consisting of handling all logistical aspects of the conference with the California Endowment Center in downtown Los Angeles, where the event is held. Preparing for the first conference was one of the most stressful yet rewarding experiences of my life. I remember my first meeting with the coordinator at the Endowment Center and her fascination as I explained to her that the purpose of SCRIPT was to provide free community intervention training and raise awareness about integrating the efforts of multiple agencies and organizations to support the public need for mental health care, crisis intervention, and supportive services in Los Angeles.

At the end of our meeting, the coordinator told me how amazing SCRIPT was for not only offering a free community conference, but also for focusing on male survivors. She was unaware of the high rates of the trauma that men in our communities are experiencing. It was in that moment that I understood why I was so attracted to SCRIPT. I realized that my father was a male survivor and how significantly his trauma had affected our relationship.

Being a part of the SCRIPT team for the past three years has not only helped me grow professionally, but it has significantly impacted me personally. I have had the opportunity to work with incarcerated men, which allowed me to gain a better understanding of how many of them were survivors of abuse and trauma, and how the residual effects of that trauma influenced many of the choices they made in their lives. I have also had the opportunity to speak with many of the attendees during the conferences. They have frequently told me how courageous SCRIPT is to publicly address the often ignored issues related to male survivors. This enormous amount of positive feedback has only fueled my passion for SCRIPT.

In the African-American community that I grew up in, mental health and trauma were rarely, if ever, discussed. The great majority of the people rely heavily on their religious beliefs and spirituality to help them work through and overcome their problems or challenges. In addition, there is often a stigma attached to mental health and to those who receive mental health services. Many individuals are unaware of the mental health resources that are available to them in their communities.

One of the main goals of SCRIPT is to involve as many community mental health organizations as we can in an effort to introduce them to the community so that individuals know they exist. By raising awareness and educating the community about the benefits of mental health services, particularly those dealing with trauma, we can end the stigma and shame that is associated with needing and seeking mental health services. The possibilities of SCRIPT, I believe, are endless. For far too long, mental health has been ignored in our communities. However, SCRIPT is striving to bridge the gap between individuals and available resources with the goal of improving the overall quality of life in our communities.

Part Two

Crystal Flores
The Chicago School of Professional Psychology
Psy.D. Student

Associate Director of Programing
SCRIPT Conference

For my dear friend.

I should start by saying that I don't believe in coincidences. Or rather, I believe that everything happens for a reason. I first heard of SCRIPT during my second year of graduate school. Dr. Warner, my professor at the time, announced to the class that she was working on a community project and she was searching for a team to help her. If anyone was interested, they could email her their curriculum vitae. Although I didn't really know what the project entailed, it was community-oriented and presented an opportunity for growth. That was enough for me. I sent my CV right after class and Dr. Warner called me for an interview. I learned that our small team, three students plus Dr. Warner, would be planning and hosting a free community conference on male survivors of trauma and abuse. I thought, *This is where the universe wants me to be. This is an important part of my journey.*

In the beginning Dr. Warner's ideas and methods seemed a little crazy, and I would be lying if I said I never asked myself, *Why the heck am I doing this again?* but I kept the faith. I knew I was playing an important role in something bigger, perhaps the start of my own professional career.

Initially I thought my interest in working on SCRIPT was due to my own background. My mom comes from a family of eight children in which abuse was common, including alcoholism, domestic violence, and physical, verbal, emotional and sexual abuse. Of the six boys, four suffered sexual abuse, and all witnessed domestic violence and alcoholism. Some of them went on to perpetrate other family members. Instead of anger, I have compassion and a passion to learn more about their story and the effects of exposure to violence and abuse on the brain.

I realized that everything in my life leading up to that point was somehow tied to male survivors of trauma – from my personal experiences, to the psychology class I took in high school, to my internship site, to the loss of a dear friend. That is probably why I decided to continue working on the conference with Dr. Warner and my colleagues, who also became my friends.

One day, I walked into Dr. Warner's office shortly before one of our biweekly meetings and sat on her red leather couch. She immediately noticed the overwhelmed and defeated look on my face, and asked me how I was doing. I proceeded to tell her my dilemma. My husband and I had lost one of our best friends in a motorcycle accident about seven months earlier. Along with the loss of our friend, we were also left with the debt of his motorcycle. Dr. Warner said, "So, why are you stressing? The money will get paid off. You will figure it out so stop stressing about it." She ultimately proved to be right.

Fast forward to 2017. I was finally mourning the loss of our friend and seeking closure. In the midst of this process I began to retrieve memories and openly discuss our friend's history. I quickly found myself connecting the dots and realized that he, too, was a survivor. His father was an alcoholic and extremely abusive toward him and his mother. My friend directly witnessed domestic violence and eventually began to defend his mom, resulting in frequent fights with his father. During the 26 years of his life, he suffered a great deal, mostly in silence. He found solace in the company of his best friend, but he was always searching for love. He was unable to find it because of the early childhood trauma that affected his behavior, mood, and relationships with people. He frequently asked for my opinion, saying that he respected me because I was going to school and reading books on psychology. He also said that he admired me for helping kids in my job at an emergency teen shelter. After I co-signed the motorcycle loan for him, he said, "Thank you for believing in me, for trusting me. Only one other person has ever believed in me, a teacher from high school. That means so much to me. I promise I will not screw you over." It was one of the last things he said to me. I now know that this was a huge reason why I continued working on SCRIPT for nearly three years.

They were busy years. I was collecting data for my dissertation, applying for practicums and internships, working at practicum sites, and completing coursework. Each year I learned more about myself through my experiences and did not realize how many new skills I had acquired while working on SCRIPT, both personally and professionally. The first year was challenging. Planning and coordinating the conference involved learning a whole new skill set. While my job was primarily administrative, my communication and social skills were also put to the test. My task involved contacting presenters, gathering biographies and abstracts for the schedule, and creating the schedule. I had no idea the task would be so tedious and result in a document that was well over 50 pages long. I also had to respond to the emails and phone calls of guests registering to attend. It was hectic and time consuming.

One day Dr. Warner and I were going back and forth trying to finalize the schedule. My husband and I had just moved and had no internet access so I had to go to Starbucks to use the WiFi. I had just left the coffee shop when Dr. Warner sent me back the document for more edits. I was embarrassed but I finally got the courage to tell her of my situation. She said, "Why didn't you say something?!" It was another moment in which I realized the importance of communication and not being afraid of disappointing or looking stupid.

This was only one of many incidents in which I was challenged to improve my weaknesses and build new skills. During my time working on SCRIPT, I learned how to plan a conference from start to finish. I also learned things like how long it can take to get responses to emails, how to work with people who have big egos, and most importantly, the power of bringing people together. At the closing ceremony, I took the time to survey the room. Police officers, SWAT team members, ex-gang members, survivors, professors, lawyers, and public figures of all ages and ethnicities had come together to collaborate on tackling issues related to male survivors of trauma and abuse. Then an unforgettable moment happened: an attendee stood and said that for the first time in his life he disclosed that he was a survivor during the conference. We had created a platform where people felt safe and comfortable enough to share their very personal stories. I realized that SCRIPT was worth every second of planning and effort I had put into it, and the beginning of something great.

I also learned more about the challenges that male survivors face: trouble with intimacy, domestic violence, and legal problems. These issues involved partners, spouses, co-workers, and family members. Providing these individuals with some form of education and support could be extremely helpful in the healing process for both the survivor and the people around him. Both parties have to deal with complexities related to everyday experiences and relationships. Learning more about survivors will ultimately help to cultivate compassion and understanding, resulting in better relationships and happiness for all.

Conclusion

Debra Warner, Psy.D.
The Chicago School of Professional Psychology
Conference Director

My goals in creating the SCRIPT conference were both personal and professional. It was created for my husband and for the community – a love letter and a resource.

Robert tells me that I don't hear him sometimes. This is a hallmark statement I've heard from many male survivors. As a spouse, maybe you can relate. Creating the SCRIPT conference was my way of telling Robert that I hear him. I don't know how to do anything on a small scale. I do everything big. It wasn't enough for me to tell him I hear him. I had to create an entire conference to tell him that. This past year was our third successful conference in a row, and it has grown into so much more than I originally envisioned.

The statement "you don't hear me" is partially accurate. Male survivors are not heard in our society. Traditional cultural masculinity demands that men be strong and rugged. They should be free of any emotion that can be perceived as feminine. And a man can't get raped. He should have been strong and defended himself. If he was raped by a woman, he must have wanted it, or even more sickening, especially in the cases where a boy is abused, he just "got lucky." No. Wrong.

Those belief systems are termites to a male survivor's psyche. They eat away at his identity, keep him from disclosing and prevent him from getting the treatment he needs. One in six boys is sexually abused in childhood. Few men disclose and receive adequate treatment. Our society pays an enormous price for not addressing this issue. How many men are lost to drug addiction, alcoholism, crime, and mental illness as a result of childhood abuse? How many children grow up with absent or emotionally distant fathers because of lack of resources? Strained relationships, divorces, violence – the list of ramifications goes on and on.

I wanted to provide a free resource for the community, to increase awareness and understanding about the issues male survivors face. This past year, I asked three presenters and two students to contribute their stories about SCRIPT. I asked them to answer: *How does SCRIPT benefit the individual?* and *how does it benefit the community?*

The first presenter I asked was Aquil Basheer, executive director and founder of the Professional Community Intervention Training Institute. Aquil and his team train and certify individuals in community-based gang outreach.

"At SCRIPT we provide individuals with the tools to change themselves. An individual who utilizes these tools, and creates change within themselves, can take that into the community and effect change. If enough individuals change, then the community changes. That is the whole concept behind what we are doing here. The blueprint we are creating for the individual is self-awareness and self-filtering. Look at your behavior and ask yourself 'Am I acting out from a place of trauma and pain? Am I communicating in an effective way? How can I communicate more effectively?'

"We teach individuals how to become 'barefoot engagers.' You can't walk into a community and simply create change. You have to take your shoes off and feel the cracks in the street, the dirt between your toes. You have to learn the culture and needs of that specific community because every community is different.

"If the only tool you're familiar with is a hammer, then every problem looks like a nail. We provide a deeper toolbox.

"The goal is normality. We want to get an individual to a baseline of normality where they can function in a comfort zone they have created for themselves by addressing their trauma. Then they can look within themselves and identify their needs and wants and begin to address those. Finally, the goal is stability and maintaining this space in the long term. If you provide temporary tools, the change is temporary. We are interested in the long term. That is how individuals become capable of changing their communities."

***

Ann Young was one of the first black women to be appointed captain in the Los Angeles Police Department. Throughout her 35-year career she tapped into the pulse of the city in her policing work. After retiring from the police department, she switched careers and is now an adjunct professor at The Chicago School of Professional Psychology.

She has spoken at every SCRIPT conference and was instrumental in planning the 2017 conference.

"The SCRIPT conference brings individuals and communities together to take a look at and address common problems. It specifically brings attention to men and male violence. There are few, if any, conferences that do what SCRIPT does. There aren't resources for men to deal with trauma, especially in the preventative stages. A lot of these men feel disconnected. There is nowhere for them to go – no place to get help. Most of the time men's issues aren't addressed until they blow up.

"Individuals change a community. When the individual changes, so will the community. The SCRIPT conference brings attention to the resources that are needed to aid individuals and the communities they are a part of."

***

Chris Anderson is a trauma theorist, survivor advocate, and a dear friend of mine. He has spoken at the SCRIPT conference each year since its creation.

"There are two unique aspects about the SCRIPT conference. First, by being a conference that brings together professionals and advocates from underserved communities, it shatters the stereotypes and barriers that prevent us from addressing trauma in society.

"Secondly, since its focus is on male victimization and male trauma, it provides a lens through which we can view trauma. Men are half of the population. It is time we start addressing the issues that affect half of our society. SCRIPT gives us that opportunity.

"We are still in a position culturally, socially, and politically where it is tough to address issues affecting men. These unaddressed issues affect our entire society."

***

What we are doing with SCRIPT is starting a movement. When I started the conference in 2015, I had no idea if it would get off the ground, or where it would lead. Three years later, it is evident that our movement has legs. We have provided a desperately needed resource to individuals, communities, students, and professionals.

My hope for this book is to add depth and weight to our movement. Three years ago, there were no resources for spouses of male trauma survivors. Millions of them were like me, doing the best they could with what they had. My dream for this book is that it provides inspiration and hope to male survivors, their spouses, and society at large. Joy fills my soul at the thought of a spouse reading this and saying, *Me too. Finally someone gets it.*

By bringing attention to this issue, I hope to bring it to the national foreground. It is time for us to provide resources for male survivors and their families – for better families, better communities, and a better society. I hope this book will be the first of many, sparking a movement so strong that one day I can retire from the field. Until then, take care of one another, and remember, whatever you're going through – me, too.

Chapter 10 Summary

The Adverse Childhood Experiences Study and Health Effects.

Like many great discoveries, the connection between early trauma and its effects later in life was discovered by a mistake. Out of that discovery has come the Adverse Childhood Experiences Study (ACES), which helps survivors identify their level of risk for developing chronic disease and illness.

As with my husband and most survivors, the experience of abuse has long been over, but its effects are felt for years, even decades, afterward in the survivor's risk factors for drug and alcohol abuse, obesity, heart problems, cancer, and other negative outcomes.

The ACES score helps identify a person's risk level so they can take action with their doctor. It's not yet known if we can reverse the risks, but we can at least be on the lookout for health problems in the men we love. In this chapter, Christopher Anderson explains the scientific thinking about the connection between traumatic events and the long shadow they cast.

Chapter 10

The Adverse Childhood Experiences Study and Health Effects

Christopher Anderson
Executive Director (Ret.), MaleSurvivor.org

In 1997 a doctor in Southern California did something remarkable. He made a mistake.

Dr. Vincent Felitti had, at the time, been overseeing a tremendously effective weight loss program for persons battling chronic and morbid obesity. The treatments at the obesity clinic worked. Patients were consistently losing over 100 pounds, and in some cases over 600 pounds. However, despite its proven effectiveness, the program had an unacceptably high dropout rate around 50%. Dr. Felitti was mystified. Why would patients receiving successful treatment for a life threatening condition leave the program time and time again? Something didn't make sense.

In order to try and get to the bottom of what was going wrong, Dr. Felitti interviewed hundreds of patients who had received successful treatment, then left the program and regained much of the weight they had lost. For these interviews, Dr. Felitti worked with a standardized set of questions he asked each patient. Over the course of dozens of interviews, he turned up nothing that really explained why so many patients were displaying such counter-intuitive behavior. One day, he made a mistake asking one of the questions. In an interview, Dr. Felitti explained:

"I misspoke...instead of asking, 'How old were you when you were first sexually active?' I asked, 'How much did you weigh when you were first sexually active?' The patient, a woman, answered, 'Forty pounds.'"

That moment led to a shocking admission by the patient. She had been sexually abused by her father starting when she was 4 years old. This was only the second time in Felitti's career that he had received a disclosure of incest from a victim, and it left him stunned. But it also provided him with a critically important piece of data that had not been previously accounted for: a foundational trauma in this person's life. Medical doctors simply didn't (and usually still do not) inquire if their patients had experienced abuse or trauma in the past. Through the modern lens of medical pathology, diseases are categorized and understood as dysfunctions of normal biological functions. The causes (though often murky and difficult to diagnose clearly) are physical in nature – a virus, a germ, or exposure to some kind of physical toxin like asbestos or tobacco smoke. Within this framework, trauma is only viewed as physical trauma – injuries sustained to the body as a result of external causes such as a gunshot or car accident. The role of childhood traumas – sexual abuse, or neglect, or growing up around domestic violence – were not considered to be significant contributing factors to harm later in life. If you survived the traumas of childhood, then any disease in adulthood must be linked to more contemporary causes.

Having made his "mistake," Felitti now became curious. Could this be the missing piece? Was it really possible so many of his patients at the obesity clinic had similar tales to tell if only asked? In the course of the following weeks, Felitti and his colleagues discovered many of the patients in his program did indeed report surviving experiences of many types of childhood abuse. It became clear that, at least for some patients, there was some connection between child abuse, sexual abuse, and obesity. But the reason for the connection remained mysterious. How could exposure to violence or abuse at such a young age give rise to the kinds of biological and behavioral dysfunction that these patients presented?

Soon another patient shared an insight that helped provide an explanation. A person who had been raped at age 23 and then subsequently gained over 100 pounds explained to Dr. Felitti, "Overweight is overlooked, and that's the way I need to be.[i]" It became clear that, at some level, the conceptual framework medical professionals were trained to use to analyze and treat obesity, and by extension possibly other health conditions, was flawed. Medical professionals were trained to view overeating as a disease, a pathologically unhealthy behavior likely exacerbated by improper functioning of the digestive system. Patients, however, had a radically different perspective. Upon actually being asked why they ate so much in spite of the clear and unmistakable physical consequences and health risks, many people reported that overeating was, at some deep level, a chosen strategy they employed for protection. As dangerous and unpleasant as it was to be obese, it felt better to them than the alternative – not being obese and having to cope with powerful feelings of anxiety and fear. In short, what Felitti recognized was that, when viewed from the perspective of the patients themselves, chronic overeating was not a behavioral or medical problem. Instead, becoming dangerously obese was a solution to other, deeper undiagnosed and untreated issues.

Thus, medical and behavioral professionals mistakenly labeled many dysfunctional behaviors as "problems" when these behaviors were actually poorly chosen solutions at resolving deeply rooted negative feelings. This foundational insight changed Dr. Felitti's understanding of the role trauma could play in the diseases of adulthood. However, he lacked sufficient data to convince other professionals of the critical importance early trauma played in the lives of many adults. After an early attempt to present his findings at a conference on obesity, Dr. Felitti received the following response from a colleague:

"He told me I was naïve to believe my patients, that it was commonly understood by those more familiar with such matters that these patient statements were fabrications to provide a cover explanation for failed lives!"[ii]

While such attitudes were (and still are) common among medical and behavioral clinicians, fortunately they were not universal. Soon Dr. Felitti found colleagues who wanted to collect the data that would allow us to better grasp the extent of the impact childhood trauma could have on health. Starting in 1995, Dr. Felitti, along with the assistance of Dr. Robert Anda from the Centers for Disease Control and others, identified 10 "adverse childhood experiences" – abuse (physical, emotional, sexual); neglect (physical, emotional); domestic violence in the home; mental illness in the home; substance abuse in the home; incarceration of a household member; parental separation/divorce.[iii] They then began asking thousands of patients in the Kaiser Permanente Health System, where Dr. Felitti was based, if they had experienced any of these kinds of negative events in childhood. Over the course of their study, over 17,000 people agreed to answer questions about what would be called the 10 ACES during regular medical intake interviews. What they found shocked them, and is continuing to lead to a paradigm shift in our understanding of the role early life traumas play in overall health and life expectancy.

According to their study, named the Adverse Childhood Experiences Survey (ACES), approximately 60% of the population has experienced at least one significant form of child abuse and or trauma. Perhaps most importantly, the researchers have been able to track the medical histories of the study participants over time. And it is clear, there is an undeniable link between childhood trauma and an increase in risk for a wide range of negative health outcomes.

Felitti, Anda, and others have published dozens of research articles in major peer-reviewed journals. What they have demonstrated is clear – childhood traumas are strongly correlated to negative health outcomes later in life. ACES scores are widely reported across all ages, genders, races. Of those who have an ACES score of 1 (indicating they had experienced 1 of the 10 ACES), 87% of those who had an ACES score of 1 actually had an ACES score higher than 1 (indicating that they experienced multiple types of adverse experiences in childhood). This means that the majority of people reporting at least one adverse childhood experience had multiple ACES in their past.

The research has shown strong links between ACES and many negative health outcomes including:

Smoking

Severe Obesity (BMI >/= 35)

Chronic Alcohol Use

Lack of Physical Activity

Depression

Drug Abuse

Sexual Promiscuity/Sexually Transmitted Disease

Suicidality[1]

The above list compromises what the ACES researchers listed as *Health Risk Factors for Leading Causes of Death in Adults*[4]. The data shows a clear and disturbing trend – the higher a person's ACES score, the greater their risk for having one or more of these risk factors. Over half (56%) of persons with an ACES score of 0 report none of the leading risk factors risk factors for most common causes of death, whereas even an ACES score of 1 lowers that figure to 42%. A higher ACE score is correlated with more risk factors. Of those who had ACES scores equal to or higher than 4 (meaning they survived at least 4 types of childhood trauma), only 14% showed none of the leading health risk factors for death. Perhaps the most shocking finding in the entire body of research so far is that, on average, the life expectancy of persons with ACES score of 6 or higher is 20 years shorter than persons with an ACES score of 0.

Since the initial research on ACES was published in 1998, further studies have been done in a number of states around the U.S. All show similar patterns in the data. In short, there is a strong correlation between childhood trauma and maltreatment and increased risk for a wide range of negative health outcomes later in life.

References

1. Stevens, J.E. (2012, October 3) ACES News, The-Adverse Childhood Experiences Study-The largest-most-important public health study you never heard of-began in an obesity clinic. Retrieved from https://acestoohigh.com/2012/10/03/the-adverse-childhood-experiences-study-the-largest-most-important-public-health-study-you-never-heard-of-began-in-an-obesity-clinic/
2. Ibid.
3. Ibid.
4. Felitti, V.J. et al., Relationship of Childhood Abuse and Household Dysfunction to Many of the Leading Causes of Death in Adults. *American Journal of Preventive Medicine*, Volume 14, Issue 4, 245-258.

The ACE Questionnaire

Dear Colleague:

Below is the questionnaire and a list of publications from the Adverse Childhood Experiences (ACE) Study. We are involved in analysis in the prospective arm of the study, which shows the biomedical, emotional, and economic consequences in medical care of abusive childhood experiences on average a half-century earlier. You may track future publications or read abstracts by using the free National Library of Medicine website, http://www.ncbi.nlm.nih.gov/entrez/query.fcgi and entering *Anda* or *Felitti* under 'author name.' Using Google Scholar also works very well, using *ACE Study*. Information of interest may be found at the websites www.ACEsConnection.com and at the CDC website: http://www.cdc.gov/ACE. At the latter site, abstracts may be read by clicking on titles.

Vincent J. Felitti, M.D.
VJFMDSDCA@mac.com

Finding Your ACE Score

While you were growing up, during your first 18 years of life:

Did a parent or other adult in the household often or very often...

Swear at you, insult you, put you down, or humiliate you? or

Act in a way that made you afraid that you might be physically hurt?

Yes No   If yes enter 1 _____

Did a parent or other adult in the household often or very often...

Push, grab, slap, or throw something at you?
or

Ever hit you so hard that you had marks or were injured?

Yes No   If yes enter 1 _____

Did an adult or person at least 5 years older than you ever...

Touch or fondle you or have you touch their body in a sexual way?
or

Attempt or actually have oral, anal, or vaginal intercourse with you?

Yes No   If yes enter 1 _____

Did you often or very often feel that...

No one in your family loved you or thought you were important or special?

or

Your family didn't look out for each other, feel close to each other, or support each other?

Yes   No   If yes enter 1 _____

Did you often or very often feel that...

You didn't have enough to eat, had to wear dirty clothes, and had no one to protect you?

or

Your parents were too drunk or high to take care of you or take you to the doctor if you needed it?

Yes   No   If yes enter 1 _____

Were your parents ever separated or divorced?

Yes   No   If yes enter 1 _____

Was your mother or stepmother...

Often or very often pushed, grabbed, slapped, or had something thrown at her?

or

Sometimes, often, or very often kicked, bitten, hit with a fist or hit with something hard?

or

Ever repeatedly hit at least a few minutes or threatened with a gun or knife?

Yes   No   If yes enter 1 _____

Did you live with anyone who was a problem drinker or alcoholic or who used street drugs?
Yes   No   If yes enter 1   _____

Was a household member depressed or mentally ill, or did a household member attempt suicide?
Yes   No   If yes enter 1____

Did a household member go to prison?
Yes   No   If yes enter 1   _____

Add up your "Yes" answers: ___
This is your ACE Score.

References

Felitti, V.J., Anda, R.F., Nordenberg, D., Williamson, D.F., Spitz, A.M., Edwards, V., Koss, M.P., et al. The relationship of adult health status to childhood abuse and household dysfunction. *American Journal of Preventive Medicine,* 1998; 14:245-258.Whitfield CL. Adverse Childhood Experiences and Trauma. *American Journal of Preventive Medicine, 1998*; 14:361-363.

Chapter 11 Summary

A Cultural Aspect on Male Abuse

Erin Langdon, of The Chicago School of Professional Psychology, begins this chapter by questioning the possibility of a universal definition for abuse. She follows up by presenting a question of whether or not we can impose universal penalties for abuse. She then puts forth cases from all around the world, of different cultures and societies, which participate in various forms of rites of passage that we as Westerners would almost certainly classify as abuse.

However, for these cultures, these rites of passage are pillars of their cultural heritage. These processes have been passed down through generations, and serve as a vital aspect of societies function. Many are regarded as necessary passages through which manhood is attained.

Langdon then focuses in from a worldview into our own backyard by analyzing rape in the culture of the U.S. military. What all of these cultures have in common, is the belief that these rituals are not abusive, but are a part of life.

So, is it even possible (and if so, how) to create laws that will define these practices as abuse and penalize them appropriately?

Furthermore, many parts of the world do not even acknowledge that men can be victims of interpersonal violence at the hands of women. Langdon cites examples of cultures from around the world whose domestic violence laws protect women from men, but not vice versa. Even in the United States, we have a primitive view of interpersonal violence. There still exists a strong stigma against men who come out as being abused by women.

Finally, Langdon presents a universal definition that has been applied to child maltreatment by the World Health Organization. However, this definition, its use in the foundation of law, and its application is entirely dependent on each culture and what they consider abuse.

Robert is Mexican-American, looks Caucasian, and grew up on the south side of Chicago. In his neighborhood, you had to be big and tough. Weakness was a vulnerability that would be preyed upon by someone bigger, tougher, and meaner. As a kid, he had to wear a mask that portrayed him to the world as someone that should not be messed with. He did it well; he is a big guy and can match aggression with equal or greater aggression if he needs to.

Behind closed doors he was being hurt. The mask was removed during the abuse. This goes against the groove of masculinity, especially in the culture he grew up in. According to the constructs of what it means to be a man, he failed to protect himself, and failed to live up to those norms.

These beliefs and values a culture holds have a deep effect on the individual. Society didn't protect Robert because he was a man. He should have protected himself. Those beliefs solidify in a male survivor's psyche. When he tells me that he is not heard, while it may be directed at me, it is really society who does not hear him.

Chapter 11

A Cultural Aspect on Male Abuse

Erin Langdon, M.A.
The Chicago School of Professional Psychology

Culture plays a critical role in the attitudes towards the manifestation and execution of male sexual trauma and abuse. Culture is not just the system of a society or nation, it is the group thought that belongs to organizations such as the military, family, institutions, gangs, and even like-minded individuals pursuing a goal (Stevens, 2007).

Most, if not all, the members of a culture hold to the same or similar beliefs, relate to the same images, symbols or myths. A culture has its own idiosyncratic behaviors and methods of learning, prejudices, and stereotypes. The traditions and customs dictate how children, women, and men should be treated and what their roles are within society (Stevens, 2007).

The list of cultural values and beliefs is a long one. As readers of acts of sexual abuse and trauma, rites of passage, corporal punishment that leads to serious injury, psychological and emotional battering, or neglect that causes malnutrition or even death we make judgment calls on labeling the behaviors abuse. However, culture is relevant not only to labeling the abuse but determining if the act is imperative to the people of that society, or simply an excuse for violence. The world is now more than separate nations and cultures; it is in many ways a collaboration of thoughts, actions, laws, and expected behaviors and attitudes. As members of this world, how can abuse be addressed under universal definitions, should it be addressed, and what are the effects of imposed punishment on the culture or cultural tradition of a people.

The Sambia are a tribe inhabiting the edge of the Eastern Highlands Province of Papua New Guinea. The peoples are horticultural, mountain-dwelling, hunters. It is a society that is deeply gender polarized and sexually segregated (Herdt, 1982; Neikta, n .d.). The rite of passage a boy will endure not only involves "ritualized homosexuality" and semen ingestion practices, a highly controversial practice in the world outside of Sambia, he will also be taught that women pose a threat to his manhood (Herdt, 1982; Neikta, n.d.). To the Sambia, heterosexual behavior and homosexual behavior are not in opposition to one another. The peoples consider the act of semen ingestion a stage or single sequence of events in the normal development of a male (Herdt, 1982; Neikta, n .d.). Sambias believe that boys cannot develop into men without the important substance of *jurungdu* which is found in semen. Without the semen, they cannot develop a muscular stature or attain the courage to be a powerful warrior (Herdt, 1982; Neikta, n.d.).

A 7-year-old Sambia boy has his first lesson in six stages. He will be separated from his mother and initiated into a men's cult. To begin his initiation, he will experience his first physical violation when a sharp stick of cane is jammed deep into his nostrils until blood flows freely and profusely (Neikta, n .d.). The Sambia believe this is a form of purification or cleansing the boy from any female contamination. His full indoctrination is begun when he is instructed to partake in oral sex with older warriors and swallow the semen (Neikta, n .d.). Over the next three stages, he will service the older warriors and be whipped. In the fourth stage, he is married after he is warned that women will be a danger to him and he is taught methods to repel that danger (Herdt, 1982; Neikta, n.d.). With the fifth stage, he must cause profuse bleeding in his nose each time his wife menstruates in order to cleanse himself of any pollution she may bring to his masculinity. In the final stage, or sixth stage, he must produce an offspring and keep the secrets of the cult to himself lest he be killed (Herdt, 1982; Neikta, n .d.). Many cultures will argue this process of rite of passage is inhumane and homosexual behavior but the Sambian people would say they are wrong that.

The Xhosa people of South Africa practice a rite of passage for males that is seen by them as mystical (Bullock, 2015). It is a secretive ritual to grow boys into warriors. It is intense, painful, and many times leads to the death of many young men. Al Jazeera (2013) reports that in 2012 at least 153 fatalities were reported mainly due to the botched circumcisions worsened by neglect and assault. The number

of boys injured over a four-year period, 2008 to 2012, exceeds 1,800 (Al Jazeera, 2013).

In the winter, young men (18 years of age or older) gather to go to the mountains or a place close but isolated from their village where they will become men (Al Jazeera, 2013; Bullock, 2015). They will spend months away from their families. During this time, they will undergo male circumcision with an *assegai* (spear) done by a surgeon with only the medicinal plant called *izichwe* applied to the wound to ease their pain (Bullock, 2015). No sounds of pain can be made lest they be considered cowards. Nelson Mandela wrote, "An uncircumcised Xhosa man is a contradiction in terms for he is not considered a man at all, but a boy. A boy will cry, but a man conceals his pain" (Mandela, 1994, p. 24). The circumcised boy then spends seven days in the cold without shelter, water, and little food (Al Jazeera, 2013; Bullock, 2015). This process to become a man is viewed by the outside world as cruel or abusive, but to the Xhosa it necessary for a boy to become a man. Laws are being written in South Africa to control the environment and procedures under which the boys are circumcised (Al Jazeera, 2013). Will this change a cultural tradition and reduce its meaning and relevance to the Xhosa society? Will laws even work?

Rape has been reported in the U.S. military, which is a culture unto itself with strict rules of conduct, rules of engagement, and expectations of behavior (Veterans Affairs, 2013-2015). In contradiction to this regimented culture is incidence of behavior so out of the realm of

understanding that the military appears to ignore or dismiss reports of male and female sexual assault (O'Brien, 2015). Though women's reports are taken more seriously (and there are many), it is predicted, based on reported cases, that 50% of all rapes are men on men (O'Brien, 2015). The military faces not only the seriousness of female rape, sexual assault, or harassment, but also addressing the multiple issues related to male rape or sexual trauma in the ranks. The "don't tell" mantra regarding homosexuality in the military extends to the male survivors of sexual assault (O'Brien, 2015). Male rape myths often halt the reporting of the offense, and the armed forces member is unable to get the help he needs. Myths such as "real men don't get raped" or "real men get injured fighting off the attack," makes it extremely hard for victims to report the attack or seek medical attention (O'Brien, 2015; Veterans Affairs, 2013-2015). The male victim is humiliated, embarrassed, or he will be considered gay since male-on-male sexual assault is falsely believed to only occur with homosexuals (O'Brien, 2015). The male service member also struggles with accusing anyone in his unit as he can be seen as divisive and acting inappropriately as a member of his unit (O'Brien, 2015; Veterans Affairs, 2013-2015). The impact of sexual trauma is the degradation of self as a man. Suffering from sexual trauma, these men feel that others feminize them and seek ways to prove their manhood. They go to extremes of stereotypical masculinity to regain their masculinity, such as sleeping with large numbers of women, joining outlaw biker gangs, or becoming fixated on bodybuilding (O'Brien,

2015). As stated in O'Brien, Keith, Shoemaker (2015), "cultural norms are further amplified and modified by military culture and impact male military sexual assault survivors to delay or obstruct their recovery" (p. 6).

Pakistan is one of the least tolerant countries of homosexuality. It is illegal to be so, and if you are caught and convicted, the sentence is 10 years in prison (de Lind van Wijngaarden, 2014). So how do we explain the openly abusive male sexual trauma of the boys who work as truck assistants throughout the country? It is not a hidden fact that boys are recruited to work as "truck cleaners" and part of their job is to service their drivers (de Lind van Wijngaarden, 2014). Boys as young as 12 are hired to help the drivers and learn the trade. However, as one boy states, "my *ustaad* made it clear to me in the very beginning that having sex with him will be part of my responsibilities as a truck cleaner" (de Lind van Wijngaarden, 2014. P. 14).

The boys are forced into finding work as truck cleaners by family deaths, poverty, or social issues at home that make being there unbearable (de Lind van Wijngaarden, 2014). There is little high-quality education so they opt for the road in lieu of boredom. Most of them are not prepared for the extra work load (sex). In most instances, their first experience is forced and occurs at a young age (de Lind van Wijngaarden, 2014). Yet, in an interview with victims, they did not consider this rape or homosexual behavior. Many start to enjoy the act, others to despise it, but all accept it as part of the job.

So where is society on this abuse? How can the laws be so stringent yet turn a blind eye to this activity that is blatantly bragged about by the drivers? As in many cultures, hiding heads in the sand comes from shame or dishonor for one's family, the taboo of talking about sexual issues in the open, and appearing to be a threat to the boy's masculinity. The crimes against these boys go unpunished (de Lind van Wijngaarden, 2014). However, Pakistan is not alone in both its condemnation of homosexuality or turning heads to sexual abuse of young boys (Pappas, et al., 2001). In India, where homosexuality is a taboo subject, certain social environments see adult men having sex with young boys as a viable alternative (sex object) when there are no women around (Pappas et al. 2001). They see this as sexual domination and proof of their masculinity (Pappas et al. 2001). In areas of south Asia where there are strong same-sex bonds or there is segregation of men and women, the sex act between men and male children is considered fairly innocent and not considered rape.

Violence or abuse of males is not always sexual. In domestic partnerships, most people immediately think that the victim is female. The National Center for Injury Prevention and Control of the Centers for Disease Control and Prevention released a report in 2010 called The National Intimate Partner and Sexual Violence Survey which found that 1 in 7 men within the United States has been a victim of severe physical violence or psychological aggression by a spouse or domestic partner (Hoff, 2012). This is not only an issue in the United States. In India, men are more likely to be victims of domestic violence than in any other country (Swarup, 2016). This is because the laws in India neither recognize nor acknowledge female on male violence as a crime. Legal cases in India reveal serious injuries and even death, yet the justice system has no penal codes to prosecute the women (Swarup, 2016).

The problem for men who are victims of intimate partner abuse, regardless of country or culture, is overcoming both the lack legal protection and social stigma (Hoff, 2012; Swarup, 2016). Cultural values and belief lead to the misguided definition and expectations of masculinity, which include being invulnerable to domestic violence. (Hoff, 2012; Swarup, 2016) A woman could not possibly inflict harm on a man, especially her domestic partner. Societies and cultures fail to be sympathetic and tend to ridicule men who are abused, rather than find answers (Hoff, 2012; Swarup, 2016). These barriers create a greater wall of silence hiding behind pride and fear. Men do not safely emerge from domestic abuse. Research is showing that they experience significant psychological trauma. This psychological trauma manifests as post-traumatic stress disorder (PTSD), depression, and often suicidal thoughts (Hoff, 2012).

Making boys into men via violence seems to be a theme in non-Western countries (and in some cultures within the U.S.). In South Sudan, Yemen, Uganda, Myanmar, Colombia, and the Eastern Democratic Republic of Congo, boys are recruited, kidnapped, or threatened to serve as soldiers for one side or the other. The total number of child soldiers is not clearly recorded, but it is estimated to be around 300,000 in 30 conflicts around the world (Bartoloni, 2012). They are forced to join the "army" where they are used as sexual objects or cannon fodder, then discarded when no longer valuable to the cause (Bartoloni, 2012). From the time of a boy's recruitment, he is subjected to a level of physical, psychological, and emotional abuse that few people could tolerate without acquiescing to the demands of the enlisters. "When they came to my village, they asked my older brother whether he was ready to join the militia. He was just 17 and he said no; they shot him in the head. Then they asked me if I was ready to sign, so what could I do - I didn't want to die" (Allen, 2006). As child soldiers, these children have the distinction of being both victim and violator, including but not limited to murder and rape. Leaders held the boys in line with threats of beatings ". . . if you slept while on watch or if you disobey, you will be bound hands and feet and beaten to death" (Trenholm, Olsson, Blomqvist, & Ahlberg, 2013, p. 10). Other forms of masculinity-making included deprivation of sleep and food, mind-altering substances, and long imposed marches (many times barefoot). Boys being made into soldiers in these cultures was a training based on the sheer will to survive; "kill or be killed" did not just apply to your enemy, but to your fellow soldiers and commanders if you stood defiant to their authority or broke rank. If a child were ordered to murder his best friend, a family member, or enemy and did not comply, he himself would be killed by his own group. (Trenholm, Olsson, Blomqvist, & Ahlberg, 2013, p. 10).

The mental, physical, and emotional recovery for boys who are finally rescued or who voluntarily leave are momentous. These boys have seen beatings or torture, violent death, stabbings, chopping, and shooting close-up. They have been beaten by armed forces, witnessed large-scale massacres, and forced to kill (Drexler, 2011). Trauma, PTSD, depression and many other mental health issues drown these children in anguish. They are usually unwelcomed back in their village because of atrocities they participated in or fear from the village of retribution from "army" or rebels (Dexter, 2011).

The World Health Organization, a strong advocate for the rights of children and stopping maltreatment gives us an international or global definition of child maltreatment:

"Child maltreatment is the abuse and neglect that occurs to children under 18 years of age. It includes all types of physical and/or emotional ill-treatment, sexual abuse, neglect, negligence, and commercial/other exploitation, which results in actual or potential harm to the child's health, survival, development or dignity in the context of a relationship of responsibility, trust or power. Exposure to intimate partner violence is also sometimes included as a form of child maltreatment." Yet the laws to curtail violations of human rights seem to be dependent on culture and the acceptance or non-acceptance of universal law.

Clearly, the world focuses on children because we are protective of the vulnerable. Perhaps, applying this definition across age and gender will help curtail blatant acts of aggression that are for financial, emotional, physical, sexual, or psychological gain of the perpetrator. As noted in previous chapters, these are not easy topics for males to confront, regardless of their ethnicity, sexual orientation, age, or culture.

References

Veterans Affairs. (2013-2015). *Military culture: Core competencies for healthcare professionals (Military organization and roles).* Department of Veterans Affairs, Employee Education System and Department of Defense.

Al Jazeera. (2013, January 01). *Ndiyindoda: I am man.* Retrieved from Al Jazeera People and Power: http://www.aljazeera.com/programmes/peopleandpower/2013/01/20131211736199557.html

Allen, K. (2006, July 25). *Bleak future for Congo's child soldiers.* Retrieved from BBC: http://news.bbc.co.uk/2/hi/africa/5213996.stm

Banyard, P. &. (2011). *Ethical issues in psychology.* New York, New York: Routledge, Inc.

Bartoloni, A. (2012, December 13). *Enduring scars: Child soldiers and mental health.* Retrieved from Irish forum for Global Health: http://globalhealth.ie/2012/12/13/enduring-scars-child-soldiers-and-mental-health/

Bullock, R. (2015, May 29). *A month with three initiates during the Xhosa circumcision ritual.* Retrieved from Africa Geographical Magazine: http://magazine.africageographic.com/weekly/issue-48/xhosa-circumcision-ritual-south-africa-its-hard-to-be-a-man/#sthash.4NvIcfjn.dpuf

de Lind van Wijngaarden, J. W. (2014). 'Part of the job': male-to-male sexual experiences and abuse of young men working as 'truck cleaners' along the highways of Pakistan. *Culture, Health & Sexuality, 16*(5), 562-574.

Drexler, M. (2011). Life after death: Helping former child soldiers become whole again. *Harvard School of Public Health.*

Galovski, T., & Lyons, J. A. (2004). Psychological sequelae of combat violence: A review of the impact of PTSD on the veteran's family and possible interventions. *Aggression and Violent Behavior,* 477-501.

Hanson, R. (2013). Hardwiring happiness: The new brain science of contentment, calm, and confidence. New York: Harmony Books.

Henry, S. B., Smith, D. B., Archuleta, K. L., Sanders-Hahs, E., Nelson Goff, B. S., Reisbig, K. L., et al. (2011). Trauma and couples: Mechanisms in dyadic functioning. *Journal of Marital and Family Therapy,* 319-332.

Herdt, G. (1982). *Rituals of manhood: Male initiation in Papua New Guinea.* Berkeley, CA: University of California Press.

Hoff, B. H. (2012, February 12). *National Study: More men than women victims of intimate partner physical violence, psychological aggression.* Retrieved from Stop Abusive and Violent Environments : http://www.saveservices.org/2012/02/cdc-study-more-men-than-women-victims-of-partner-abuse/

Meis, L. A., Kehle, S. M., Barry, R. A., Erbes, C. R., & Polusny, M. A. (2010). Relationship adjustment, PTSD symptoms, and treatment utilization among coupled

National Guard soldiers deployed to Iraq. *Journal of Family Psychology*, 560-567.

Neikta. (n.d.). *Sambia Tribe's initiation from boyz to men.* Retrieved from Orijin Culture: http://www.orijinculture.com/community/masculini sation-dehumanization-sambia-tribe-papua-guinea/

O'Brien, C. K. (2015). Don't tell: Military culture and male rape. *Psychological Services, 12*(4), 357–365.

Pappas, G. K. (2001). "Males who have sex with males (MSM) and HIV/AIDS in India: The hidden epidemic. *AIDS and Public Policy Journal, 16*(1), 4-17.

Schnarch, D. (2009). Passionate marriage: Keeping love and intimacy alive in committed relationships. New York: W.W. Norton & Co.

Stevens, M. J. (2007). Toward a global psychology: Theory, research, intervention, and pedagogy. . Mahwah, NJ: Lawrence Erlbaum Associates, Inc.

Swarup, S. (2016, October 11). *Domestic violence against men.* Retrieved from merinews: http://www.merinews.com/article/domestic-violence-against-men/15920158.shtml

Taft, C. T., Stafford, J., Watkins, L. E., & Street, A. E. (2011). Posttraumatic stress disorder and intimate relationship problems: A meta-analysis. *Journal of Consulting and Clinical Psychology*, 22-33.

Trenholm, J. O. (2013, January 16). Constructing soldiers from boys in Eastern Democratic Republic of Congo. *Men and Masculinities, 16*(2), 203-227.

Van der Kolk, B. (2014). The body keeps score: Brain, mind, and body in the healing of trauma. New York: Penguin.

Van der Kolk, B., McFarlane, A. C., & Weisaeth, L. E. (1996). Traumatic stress: The effects of overwhelming experience on mind, body, and society. New York: Guilford.

Chapter 12 Summary

Extended Family – They Won't Get It

Disbelief, minimizing, and denial are the most common reactions by family members when a disclosure is made by a survivor of abuse. It's commonplace for parents to ignore the signs in their children, the change in personality, school performance, or weight gain. The effects that are so obvious in retrospect – the low self-esteem, the depression, the sense of shame – go unaddressed by the family because no one wants to believe that a child could be abused by someone in their close family circle – it's the "stranger danger" that we are all warned about.

But the truth is that most abuse is within the family or close family circle. That's what happened to my husband.

When he finally did disclose to his mother, years after the event happened, her first reaction was to minimize it, "Are you sure it wasn't just kids playing?" It's not acceptable to support the minimization, but we do need to understand that it will happen. Family will instinctively "close ranks" and question if the abuse was really abuse. As spouses we need to recognize when a disclosure is happening. Simply acknowledging it to our husbands or partners is hugely empowering and validating to them.

Men are scared to admit the abuse in the first place and they're scared of the reactions, therefore they will delay as long as possible talking about it. Whatever we can do to make it OK for them is crucial to their healing.

Chapter 12

Extended Family – They Won't Get It

Jennifer Harman, Ph.D.
Colorado State University

Survivors of trauma resulting from childhood abuse (in its many forms) face challenges in their close family and intimate relationships. Many survivors struggle with internalizing mental health problems such as depression (Lowe & Balfour, 2015) and anxiety (Grossman, Spinazzola, Zucker, & Hopper, 2017), shame, and low self-esteem, all of which make it difficult to talk to others about their abuse experience (Lowe, Willan, Kelly, Hartwell, & Canuti, 2016).

The needs of adult survivors of psychological abuse, emotional maltreatment, and neglect are even less poorly known than other forms of abuse (e.g., sexual; Grossman, Spinazzola, Zucker, & Hopper, 2017). These survivors tend to show greater impairments in their ability to form and maintain healthy relationships, and use less adaptive coping strategies to deal with their experience, such as engaging in greater amounts of self-injury (e.g., cutting) and substance abuse than those with other forms of abuse, particularly male survivors (e.g., Cross, Crow, Powers, &

Bradley, 2015). Although influential relationships such as family and intimate partners can provide social support which can serve as turning points for male survivors to have healthier trajectories in their lives (Easton, Leone-Sheehan, Sophis, & Willis, 2015), trust issues that evolved due to relational injuries experienced as youth make it difficult for survivors to feel safe in their adult relationships (Wells, Lobo, Galick, Knudson-Martin, Huenergardt, & Schaepper, 2017).

Unfortunately, many extended family members and intimate partners do not understand the needs of the adult male abuse survivor. Survivors do not often disclose the legacy of their childhood abuse until adulthood out of fear of being blamed or shunned by family members for their experience (Davies, Patel, & Rogers, 2013). Many disclosures of past abuse are not believed, particularly if the target of the disclosure does not know of others who have experienced interpersonal trauma (Miller & Cromer, 2015). Some family members deny the survivor's experience altogether (e.g. Dorahy & Clearwater, 2012).

Men are less likely to disclose their history of abuse than women, and if they do, they do so much later in life (O'Leary & Barber, 2008) which can lessen the believability of their experience by others close to them (e.g. *why did it take so long for you to tell me?*). Masculine norms have been cited as one of the reasons for this lack of, or lateness in disclosure, as men are often expected to be competitive, self-reliant, in emotional control, and strong (Mahalik, Locke, Ludlow, Diemer, Scott, Gottfried, & Freitas, 2003). Being a victim of abuse is not consistent with these gender norms, so many men struggle with gender role conflicts due to their victimization (Lew, 2004). Disclosing or discussing childhood abuse conflicts with the expectation that men should have emotional control and be strong. Male survivors of sexual abuse by another man may also experience shame and fear of stigma due to homophobic attitudes shared by others in their communities (Spataro, Wells, & Moss, 2001).

Perceptions of extended family and close, intimate partners are also influenced by masculine norms and feelings. For example, norms that men should be strong may influence perceptions that men who have been abused are weak. The emotional response of the perceiver can also influence the stereotypes they have towards victims. For example, individuals who experience unpleasant affect when they learn an individual has been sexually abused (e.g., anger, nervousness, fear) evaluate survivors more negatively than when they experienced empathy for the survivor (e.g., Zafar & Ross, 2013). Because many childhood experiences of abuse occur within the family, extended family members are likely to experience negative affective responses to news of abuse, given that they have familial bonds with the perpetrator(s), as well as the survivor. Psychological abuse and neglect are not as visible forms of abuse as physical abuse, so friends and family perceive those forms of abuse as harmless or insignificant because it is not as visible as physical violence (Seff, Beaulaurier, & Newman, 2008). Due to the perceptions that the abuse is not as "serious," these individuals may not provide the survivor with the social support that they need, making the survivor believe that the family members just don't understand them.

Therapeutic interventions utilizing a family systems approach would be beneficial to facilitate greater understanding of the male survivor's needs, feelings about their experience and identity as a result of their abuse, and support communication between those close to them. Abuse is transmitted inter-generationally (Widom, 2017), so such an approach can help not only the survivor, but prevent further potential abuses within the family system.

References

Cross, D., Crow, T., Powers, A., & Bradley, B. (2015). Childhood trauma, PTSD, and problematic alcohol and substance use in low-income African-American men and women. *Child Abuse & Neglect, 44,* 26-35. doi: 10.1016/j.chiabu.2015.01.007

Davies, M., Patel, F., & Rogers, P. (2013). Examining the roles of victim-perpetrator relationship and emotional closeness in judgments toward a depicted child sexual abuse case. *Journal of Interpersonal Violence, 28,* 887–909.

Dorahy, M. J., & Clearwater, K. (2012). Shame and guilt in men exposed to childhood sexual abuse: A qualitative investigation. *Journal of Child Sexual Abuse, 21,* 155-175. doi: 10.1080/10538712.2012.659803.

Easton, S. D., Leone-Sheehan, D. M., Sophis, E. J., & Willis, D. G. (2015). 'From that moment on my life changed': Turning points in the healing process for men recovering from child sexual abuse. *Journal of Child Sexual Abuse, 24,* 152-173.

Grossman, F. K., Spinazzola, J., Zucker, M., & Hopper, E. (2017). Treating adult survivors of childhood emotional abuse and neglect: A new framework. *American Journal of Orthopsychiatry, 87,* 86-93. doi: 10.1037/ort0000225

Lew, M. (2004). Victims no longer: The classic guide for men recovering from sexual child abuse. New York, NY: Harper Perennial

Lowe, M., & Balfour, B. (2015). The unheard victims. *The Psychologist, 28,* 118–124.

Lowe, M., Willan, V. J., Kelly, S., Hartwell, S., & Canuti, E. (2016). CORE assessment of adult survivors abused as children: A NAPAC group therapy evaluation. *Counseling & Psychotherapy Research, 17,* 71-79. doi: 10.1002/capr.12095

Mahalik, J. R., Locke, B. D., Ludlow, L. H., Diemer, M. A., Scott, R. P. J., Gottfried, M., & Freitas, G. (2003). Development of the conformity to masculine norms inventory. *Psychology of Men and Masculinity, 4,* 3–25.

Miller, K. E., & Cromer, L. D. (2015). Beyond gender: Proximity to interpersonal trauma in examining differences in believing child abuse disclosures. *Journal of Trauma & Dissolution, 16,* 211-223.

O'Leary, P. J., & Barber, J. (2008). Gender differences in silencing following childhood sexual abuse. *Journal of Child Sexual Abuse, 17,* 133-143. doi: 10.1080/10538710801916416

Seff, L. R., Beaulaurier, R. L., & Newman, F. L. (2008). Nonphysical abuse: Findings in domestic violence against older women study. *Journal of Emotional Abuse, 8,* 355–374.

Spataro, J., Moss, S. A., & Wells, D. L. (2001). Child sexual abuse: A reality for both sexes. *Australian Psychologist, 36,* 177–183.

Wells, M. A., Lobo, E., Galick, A., Knudson-Martin, C., Huenergardt, D., & Schaepper, H. (2017). Fostering trust through relational-safety: Applying socio-emotional relationship therapy's focus on gender and power with heterosexual adult-survivor couples. *Journal of Couple &*

Relationship Therapy, 16, 122-145. doi:10.1080/15332691.2016.1238795

Widom, C. S. (2017). Long-term impact of child abuse and neglect on crime and violence. *Clinical Psychology,* online first publication. doi: 10.1111/cpsp.12194

Zafar, S., & Ross, E. C. (2013). Perceptions of childhood sexual abuse survivors: Development and initial validation of a new scale to measure stereotypes of adult survivors of childhood sexual abuse. *Journal of Child Sexual Abuse, 22,* 358-378. doi: 10.1080/10538712.2013.743955

Chapter 13 Summary

Male Trauma Survivors in the LGBTQ Community

This chapter addresses the specialized concerns and issues of men (both biological gender and transgender) in the Lesbian, Gay, Bisexual, Transgender, and Queer (LGBTQ) community who are facing a host of traumas, from Inter-Personal Violence (IPV) to societal intolerance and institutional discrimination, harassment and even abuse.

For members of the LGBTQ community, the thread of trauma runs through their lives linking family intolerance and/or abusive responses to coming out, to partner abuse in the forms of emotional, mental, and financial control. As a minority group within the community of men who have been abused, the gay, bisexual and trans man has additional opportunities to experience trauma in the form of internalized homophobia, externalized homophobia from society and even from those whom he turns to for protection – the police and domestic violence shelters.

As my husband has shared, it's difficult to disclose under the best of circumstances when the perpetrator is another man because there are the increased concerns of being labeled as homosexual or bisexual. When a survivor reaches out to the police, incidents of homophobia can manifest in derogatory language, disbelief, and sometimes further abuse by the demand for sexual favors in exchange for protection. Domestic violence shelters are not always properly trained or properly equipped to handle LGBTQ survivors.

For LGBTQ men who are of color or immigrants, there is an even deeper level of potential trauma involved in being a minority within a minority within a minority. The best way that we can reduce continuing harm is to educate the service providers. We do that by speaking about the abuse. Whether the survivor is homosexual, bisexual, transgendered or a biologically gendered heterosexual, we must shine the light on the problem to fix it.

Chapter 13

Male Trauma Survivors in the LGBTQ Community

Adam F. Yerke, Psy.D.
Ashley Fortier, M.A.
The Chicago School of Professional Psychology

As demonstrated throughout this book, male trauma survivors are frequently hidden in the shadows of female survivors. Male trauma survivors of the Lesbian, Gay, Bisexual, Transgender, and Queer (LGBTQ) community are recognized even less. This chapter brings to light the experiences of male trauma survivors who identify as gay, bisexual, transgender, and/or queer. The types of trauma experienced by this group are distinct from heterosexual and cisgender (non-transgender) people as indicated by the preponderance of hate crimes, specific intimate partner violence tactics, persistent minority stress, and harmful interactions with law enforcement when seeking help. Consequently, mental health and intimate relationships for male survivors of the LGBTQ community are impacted uniquely. Enhanced understanding of this topic encourages improved prevention and intervention efforts for male survivors of the LGBTQ community, thereby promoting healing for afflicted individuals and their relationships.

This chapter focuses on male survivors of the LGBTQ community, including gay, bisexual, transgender, and queer identified men. However, it's necessary to consider the limitations of grouping these individuals together, given the diversity within and between each of these specific populations. When possible, the distinction is at least made between sexual orientation and gender identity, therefore differentiating people who are gay, bisexual, or queer versus transgender. Also, the reader should consider that individuals often take on multiple identities, such as identifying as transgender and bisexual. Moreover, identities referred to by the acronym LGBTQ does not reflect all terms used by this broader community, particularly as new ways to define one's sexual orientation and gender identity continue to emerge. Finally, information given about transgender survivors is not specific to transgender men and must be regarded carefully, given the disproportionate rates of trauma among transgender women.

Hate-Based Violence

Trauma can occur for LGBTQ people in many of the same ways as for heterosexual and cisgender people. However, LGBTQ people are additionally targeted because of bias against their sexual orientation and/or gender identity. In 2015, roughly 18% of all bias-related crimes were motivated by sexual orientation, and nearly 2% of the 7,173 victims were targeted on the basis of gender identity. (Federal

Bureau of Investigation [FBI], 2016). This type of violence, referred to as hate-based, includes physical violence, verbal harassment, sexual violence, and discrimination (National Coalition of Anti-Violence Programs [NCAVP], 2016a). In a recent study of 1,250 LGBTQ survivors, participants who endorsed experiences of hate-based violence cited the types they experienced: verbal harassment (15%), discrimination (14%), physical violence (12%), and threats or intimidation (11%) (NCAVP, 2016a). Hate-based violence directed at LGBTQ people tends to be more violent, involve multiple perpetrators, and result in more severe injuries, when compared to violent crimes not committed due to bias (Stotzer, 2016a).

Hate-based violence is especially common for certain LGBTQ groups. Gay men are the most targeted, even when considering all other crimes motivated by biases, such as religion or ethnicity (FBI, 2010; Herek, 2009). Even compared to lesbian and bisexual women, gay and bisexual men are at increased risk of hate-based violence (Stotzer, 2016a). For instance, research showed that the majority of LGBTQ people who endure hate-based violence identified as gay (47%) compared to lesbian (17%) or heterosexual (14%) (NCAVP, 2016a). Risk and severity of hate-based violence further increase when LGBTQ people are other than White. Of those who experienced hate-based violence, LGBTQ people of color were twice as likely as white LGBTQ people to experience physical violence (NCAVP, 2016a). Immigration status also contributes to risk, as undocumented LGBTQ people were four times as likely to experience physical violence (NCAVP, 2016a).

Transgender people are also more likely to recall hate-based violence. In a recent study of 27,715 participants, transgender people reported experiences of verbal harassment (46%) and physical violence (14%) (James, Herman, Rankin, Keisling, Mottet, & Anafi, 2016). Specific to sexual violence, nearly half (47%) of participants reported having been sexually assaulted, and one out of ten participants (10%) had been sexually assaulted in the past year (James et al., 2016). Hate-based crimes against transgender people tend to involve perpetration by strangers, consist of multiple perpetrators, and be more violent, even compared to hate-based crimes against gay men (Stotzer, 2016a). In addition, transgender people frequently experience hate-based violence multiple times (Stotzer, 2016a, p. 1245).

Intimate Partner Violence

Trauma may also occur for LGBTQ people due to intimate partner violence (IPV). A review of relevant research showed that of men who had experienced IPV, the majority were bisexual (37.3%), followed by heterosexual (28.7%) and gay (25.2%) (Brown & Herman, 2015). This suggests that men, regardless of their sexual orientation, are not immune to IPV, and this is a frequent issue for gay and bisexual men. In a study of 1,976 LGBTQ IPV survivors, the most common types of IPV cited were: physical violence (20%), verbal harassment (18%), and threats and intimidation (13%) (NCAVP, 2016b).

Consistent with information about hate-based violence, marginalized LGBTQ people are more vulnerable to IPV, including people of color, undocumented immigrants, individuals with disabilities, and transgender people (NCAVP, 2016b). Transgender people suffer alarming rates of IPV as indicated by a recent study where more than half of participants (54%) expressed having experienced some form of IPV (James et al., 2016). In addition, 24% had experienced "severe physical violence" by a partner compared to 18% in the general population (James et al., 2016, p. 13).

Gay and Bisexual Men

Gay and bisexual men experience IPV in many of the same ways as heterosexual men such as through verbal, emotional, physical, sexual, or economic abuse as well as stalking (Rothman & Nnawulezi, 2016). More specifically, Rothman and Nnawulezi (2016) reported that the U.S. National Intimate Partner and Sexual Violence Survey (NISVS) found that 26% of gay men and 37% of bisexual men had experienced physical violence, rape, and/or stalking within an intimate relationship compared to 29% of heterosexual men. In addition, multiple researchers have found that gay and bisexual men are more vulnerable to higher severity of physical injury compared to heterosexual men (Kuehnle & Sullivan, 2003; Merrill & Wolfe, 2000; Batholomew, Regan, White & Oram, 2008).

Beyond the typical forms of IPV, gay and bisexual men often endure additional abusive tactics based on their sexual orientation (Rothman & Nnawulezi, 2016). For instance, an abuser may exert power and control by threatening to "out" their partner – that is, disclose the partner's sexual orientation to others without consent. An abuser may additionally minimize and deny actions as abusive, explaining that IPV does not exist in same-sex relationships. Alternatively, an abuser may challenge his partner's sexual orientation by questioning whether they are "really" gay or bisexual. Abusers can also monopolize resources, such as reporting to friends and/or service providers that they are the "real" victim.

In some cases, each partner can be both a victim and perpetrator, referred to as bidirectional abuse. The consequences can be especially severe when this dynamic occurs since abuse tends to escalate when both partners act aggressively (Capaldi, Kim & Shortt, 2004; Ehrensaft, Moffit, Caspi, 2004; Landolt & Dutton, 1997). In addition, gay and bisexual men frequently encounter problems when seeking support services due to providers' difficulty differentiating between abuser and victim (Batholomew, Regan, White & Oram, 2008).

Transgender People

Transgender people also experience the same types of IPV (physical, emotional, sexual, and/or financial) as cisgender people. However, when cisgender individuals are abusive towards their transgender partners in the context of a relationship, they tend to utilize vulnerabilities unique to being transgender to exert their power and control (Brown, 2011; Yerke & DeFeo, 2016). Just as with IPV among gay and bisexual men, the abuser may threaten to "out" their partner by disclosing their gender identity or birth-assigned sex to others (FORGE, 2011; White & Goldberg, 2006). In addition, abuse often includes increased focus on gender-specific body features such as chests and genitals. For instance, abusive partners may insult aspects of their transgender partner's body which bring them discomfort (FORGE, 2011), and such features may be directly targeted during physical violence (White & Goldberg, 2006). An abusive partner may also commit financial abuse by withholding money necessary for transgender-specific medical services such as hormones or surgery as well as items used for expressing their gender identity, such as clothing (FORGE, 2011; White & Goldberg, 2006).

Minority Stress

Trauma experienced by LGBTQ people encompasses more than overt violence. In a study of 2,283 LGBTQ people, the vast majority (74%) reported having experienced prejudice or discrimination related to sexual orientation and/or gender identity (Kaiser Family Foundation, 2001). For example, LGBTQ people report persistent discrimination related to employment, housing, healthcare, and public accommodation (e.g. hotels, restaurants, and public transportation). In addition, laws are not always in place to protect LGBTQ people from discrimination as with other marginalized groups. And even where anti-discrimination laws exist, they are not always enforced. The more that individuals encounter discrimination for being

LGBTQ, the more physical and psychological consequences they suffer (Meyer, 2003; Whitman & Nadal, 2016)

Being persistently discriminated against due to stigma associated with sexual orientation and/or gender identity generates unique stress for LGBTQ people, referred to as minority stress (Meyer, 2003). A consequence to this phenomenon is that LGBTQ people are more likely to develop physical and mental health problems, especially anxiety, depression, post-traumatic stress disorder (PTSD), panic disorder, suicidality, and substance abuse (Whitman & Nadal, 2016). In addition, minority stress is even more pronounced for marginalized people within the LGBTQ community, including people of color, those with disabilities, undocumented immigrants, and transgender people.

Comprehending the magnitude of minority stress for LGBTQ people requires recognition that society tends to value heterosexual and cisgender identities and marginalizes sexual and gender-based minorities. LGBTQ people continually receive messages that being other than heterosexual and cisgender makes them inferior, referred to as microaggressions (Whitman & Nadal, 2016). These attacks to LGBTQ people range from being purposeful to unconscious by the aggressor. For instance, using derogatory language to insult someone because of being gay is understandably harmful. However, less conspicuous microaggressions, like indicating that all gay men have effeminate mannerisms, are just as damaging. In fact, the constant surge of microaggressive attacks may prove to be just as traumatic for LGBTQ people as experiences of violence.

Law Enforcement

Despite the pervasiveness of trauma, LGBTQ people commonly decide against seeking assistance from law enforcement. For instance, in a recent study, only 41% of LGBTQ people indicated they reported their experiences of hate violence to police (NCAVP, 2016a). Of those who sought assistance by law enforcement, 41% said that police responded indifferently and 39% said they were hostile. Of participants who reported negative police behavior, they encountered verbal abuse (33%), physical violence (16%), the use of slurs or biased language against them (8%), and sexual violence (3%). With regard to IPV, 43% of LGBTQ participants reported interacting with law enforcement because of IPV, but only 33% made a formal report (NCAVP, 2016b). Of those who interacted with law enforcement, participants described police as hostile (12%) and indifferent (13%), and reported misarrests of survivors occurred (31%).

Transgender people have been even more perturbed by their interactions with law enforcement, thus dissuading them from seeking help with trauma. In a recent study, James et al. (2016) reported 57% of participants said they would feel uncomfortable asking police for help if they needed it. In the past year, 58% of participants had interacted with police, and of this group, the following types of mistreatment were described: repeated use of wrong gender pronouns (49%), verbal harassment (20%), officers asked questions about gender transition (19%), officers assumed they were sex workers (11%), physically attacked (4%), sexually assaulted by officers (3%), and forced to engage in sexual activity to avoid arrest (1%). Because of their negative experiences, LGBTQ people may run the risk of future victimization by avoiding police contact.

Mental Health

The effects of trauma are devastating for anyone. However, LGBTQ people are already more vulnerable to physical and psychological health problems as a result of minority stress. For instance, LGBTQ people are three times more likely to experience a mental health condition (National Alliance on Mental Illness [NAMI], 2016). In addition, substance abuse is more frequent, as 20% to 30% of LGBTQ people abuse substances, compared to 9% of the general population (NAMI, 2016). The transgender population is identified as faring even worse and it's estimated that between 38% and 65% of have experienced suicidal ideation (NAMI, 2016).

When exposed to trauma, the most common consequences for LGBTQ people include: increased suicidality, post-traumatic stress disorder (PTSD) symptoms, depression, substance use, and decreased trust of others and of a just world (Sotzer, 2016b). Specific to gay and bisexual men, trauma survivors most commonly experience: depression, anxiety, PTSD symptoms, eating disorders, substance use, academic problems, sexually transmitted infections (STIs), injuries, and death (Rothman

& Nnawulezi, 2016). The most common consequences for transgender survivors include: suicidality, depression, substance use, PTSD symptoms, sexual risk-taking, HIV risk, and mental health complaints (Stotzer, 2016c).

Intimate Relationships

Trauma widely impacts people's lives, including their intimate relationships. For gay, bisexual, and queer male survivors, their abilities to form relationships tend to be negatively impacted as noted by difficulties in their relationships and more frequent termination of relationships (Stotzer, 2016b, p. 1058). Gay, bisexual, and queer men also experience hate-based violence because of bias against their sexual orientation; therefore, given that their intimate relationships relate to their trauma, there is additional pressure associated with being together. Simply being in a relationship with one another may add to the frequency and types of discrimination they experienced.

How relationship difficulties manifest may be similar to that of heterosexual relationships where one or both partners have experienced trauma. For instance, trauma often leads to the development of distorted cognitions which affect perceptions of one's personal identity, others, safety, trust, self-esteem, control, and intimacy. The altering of perceptions then leads to behavioral changes (Ponce, Williams & Allen, 2004). One such situation may be when gay, bisexual, and queer men, out of fear for their safety, decide against going out at night or showing affection to their partners in public (Stotzer, 2016b). Therefore, their engagement in the community may be restricted by having experienced trauma leading a couple to isolate and withdraw from sources of support (Stotzer, 2016b). These patterns can perpetuate mental health symptoms associated with trauma and minority stress. Downs (2006) further demonstrates the progression of challenges for gay, bisexual, and queer male survivors in relationships:

The presence of relationship trauma often makes it difficult, and sometimes impossible, for the sufferer to experience a satisfying relationship. He is constantly scanning the relationship environment for signs of betrayal or abuse. This expenditure of energy alone transforms a relationship from a satisfying experience into a very tiring job. As can be imagined, it's no piece of cake to live with a man who interprets even small things as relationship-destroying or who privately assumes that the relationship will not exist in the future. Sadly, the relationship trauma victim often behaves in such a way to elicit more rejection and even trauma from those around him (pp. 134-135)

Relationships involving one or both transgender people are also unique, given the stressors associated with being transgender. In response to trauma, transgender people frequently adjust their behaviors in attempt to avoid further victimization (Stotzer, 2016c). For instance, they may switch between expressing their authentic gender identity and birth-assigned gender to manage the risk of violence associated with their environment. In addition, like other survivors, transgender people may avoid going out at night and withdraw from community interactions. Consequently, such behavioral changes could result in fewer experiences of violence, but at the cost of isolation and loneliness (Stotzer, 2016c). Those in intimate relationships with transgender trauma survivors may find it difficult to cope with their partner's continuous fear and avoidance, particularly when directed at them.

Conclusion

This chapter has presented issues confronted by male trauma survivors of the LGBTQ community. For this population, trauma comes in the form of hate-based violence or discrimination, intimate partner violence, minority stress, or negative experiences with law enforcement. The consequences of trauma are different for each individual, within and beyond the LGBTQ community, but mental health and intimate relationships are among the most impacted. The complex interplay between gender, sexual orientation, trauma, and relationships merits further investigation to determine the most effective routes for prevention and intervention. In the meantime, trauma service providers (e.g. police officers and domestic violence advocates) must extend support to gay, bisexual, queer, and transgender men with respect and recognition for their unique challenges and strengths, thereby initiating the healing process.

References

Bartholomew, K., Regan, K.V., White, M.A. & Oram, D. (2008). Patterns of abuse in male same-sex relationships. *Violence and Victims. 23*(5), 617-636.

Brown, N. (2011). Holding tensions of victimization and perpetration: Partner abuse in trans communities. In J.L. Ristock's (Ed.), *Intimate partner violence in LGBTQ lives* (pp. 153-168). New York, NY: Routledge Publishing.

Brown, T.N.T. & Herman, J.L. (2015). *Intimate partner violence and sexual abuse among LGBT people: A review of existing literature.* Retrieved from https://williamsinstitute.law.ucla.edu/research/violence-crime/intimate-partner-violence-and-sexual-abuse-among-lgbt-people/

Capaldi, D.M., Kim, H.K., & Shortt, J.W. (2004). Women's involvement in aggression in young adult romantic relationships: A developmental systems model. In Putallaz, M. B. & Bierman, K. L. (Eds.), *Aggression, antisocial behavior, and violence among girls: A developmental perspective* (pp. 223–241). New York: Guilford.

Downs, A. (2006). Velvet rage: Overcoming the pain of growing up gay in a straight man's world. USA: Da Capo Press.

Ehrensaft, M.K., Moffitt, T.E., & Caspi, A. (2004). Clinically abusive relationships in an unselected birth cohort: Men's and women's participation and developmental antecedents. *Journal of Abnormal Psychology, 113,* 258–271.

Federal Bureau of Investigation (FBI). (2010). *Hate crime statistics, 2009.* Retrieved from https://www2.fbi.gov/ucr/hc2009/index.html

Federal Bureau of Investigation (FBI). (2016). *Hate crime statistics, 2015.* Retrieved from https://ucr.fbi.gov/hate-crime/2015/home

FORGE. (2011). *Transgender domestic violence and sexual assault resource sheet.* Retrieved from http://www.avp.org/storage/documents/Training% 20and%20TA%20Center/2011_FORGE_Trans_DV_SA_ Resource_Sheet.pdf

Herek, G.M. (2009). Hate crimes and stigma-related experiences among sexual minority adults in the United States. *Journal of Interpersonal Violence, 24,* 54–74. doi:10.1177/0886260508316477

James, S.E., Herman, J.L., Rankin, S., Keisling, M., Mottet, L., & Anafi, M. (2016). *The Report of the 2015 U.S. Transgender Survey.* Washington, DC: National Center for Transgender Equality.

Kaiser Family Foundation. (2001). Inside-OUT: A report on the experiences of lesbians, gays and bisexuals in America and the public's views on issues and policies related to sexual orientation. Retrieved from https://kaiserfamilyfoundation.files.wordpress.com/2 013/01/new-surveys-on-experiences-of-lesbians-gays-and-bisexuals-and-the-public-s-views-related-to-sexual-orientation-chart-pack.pdf

Kelly, C.E. & Warshafsky, L. (1987, July). *Partner abuse in gay male and lesbian couples.* Paper presented at the Third

National Conference for Family Violence Researchers, Durham, NH.

Kuehnle, K. & Sullivan, A. (2003). Gay and lesbian victimization: Reporting factors in domestic violence and bias incidents. *Criminal Justice and Behavior, 30(1)*, 85-96.

Landolt, M.A. & Dutton, D.G. (1997). Power and personality: An analysis of gay male intimate abuse. *Sex Roles*, 37, 335-359.

Merrill, G.S. & Wolfe, V.A. (2000). Battered gay men: An exploration of abuse, help seeking, and why they stay. *Journal of Homosexuality, 39*(2), 1-30. doi: 10.1300/J082v39n02_01

Meyer, I.H. (2003). Prejudice, social stress, and mental health in lesbian, gay and bisexual populations: Conceptual issues and research evidence. *Psychological Bulletin, 129*, 674-697. doi:10.1037/0033-2909.129.5.674

National Alliance on Mental Illness (NAMI). (2016). LGBTQ. Retrieved from https://www.nami.org/Find-Support/LGBTQ

National Coalition of Anti-Violence Programs (NCAVP). (2016a). *Lesbian, gay, bisexual, transgender, queer, and HIV-affected hate violence in 2015.* Retrieved from http://www.avp.org/storage/documents/ncavp_hvr eport_2015_final.pdf

National Coalition of Anti-Violence Programs (NCAVP). (2016b). *Lesbian, gay, bisexual, transgender, queer, and HIV-affected intimate partner violence in 2015.* Retrieved from http://avp.org/wp-

content/uploads/2017/04/2015_ncavp_lgbtqipvreport
.pdf

Ponce, A.N., Williams, M.K. & Allen, G.J. (2004). Experience of maltreatment as a child and acceptance of violence in adult intimate relationships: Mediating effects of distortions in cognitive schemas. *Violence & Victims,* *19*(1), 97-108. doi: 10.1891/vivi.19.1.97.33235

Rothman, E. & Nnawulezi, N. (2016). Intimate partner violence, male. In A. Goldberg (Ed.), *The SAGE Encyclopedia of LGBTQ Studies* (pp. 467-468). Thousand Oaks, CA: SAGE Publications.

Stotzer, R.L. (2016a). Hate crimes. In A. Goldberg (Ed.), *The SAGE Encyclopedia of LGBTQ Studies* (pp. 467-468). Thousand Oaks, CA: SAGE Publications.

Stotzer, R.L. (2016b). Sexual minorities and violence. In A. Goldberg (Ed.), *The SAGE Encyclopedia of LGBTQ Studies* (pp. 1055-1058). Thousand Oaks, CA: SAGE Publications.

Stotzer, R.L. (2016c). Transgender people and violence. In A. Goldberg (Ed.), *The SAGE Encyclopedia of LGBTQ Studies* (pp. 1245-1246). Thousand Oaks, CA: SAGE Publications.

White, C. & Goldberg, J. (2006). Expanding our understanding of gendered violence: Violence against trans people and their loved ones. *Canadian Women's Studies, 25*(1-2), 124-127.

Whitman, C.N. & Nadal, K.L. (2016). Microaggressions. In A. Goldberg (Ed.), *The SAGE Encyclopedia of LGBTQ*

Studies (pp. 768-770). Thousand Oaks, CA: SAGE Publications.

Yerke, A.F. & DeFeo, J. (2016). Redefining intimate partner violence beyond the binary to include transgender people. *Journal of Family Violence, 31*(8), 975-979.

Chapter 14 Summary

Effects of Childhood Trauma through the Lifespan

In this chapter Dr. Cris Ann Scaglione explains how and why trauma experienced in early childhood will continue to impact someone's life and how they operate in the world throughout their lifetime. Young children are very impressionable before they have developed a strong sense of themselves, and any traumas experienced will leave a lasting effect.

My husband's early experiences of being exposed to sexual behaviors and age-inappropriate relationships were some of the greatest influences in developing who he is and how he reacts to the world. Through a great deal of effort, he's changed how he initially responds to events today.

Nevertheless, overcoming the sense of self-doubt, the negative self-talk, and the intrusive thoughts of being a survivor is a constant struggle that has its peaks and valleys.

The patterns of emotional responses can be reshaped over time, but it is a slow and arduous process. Sometimes it takes a lifetime to identify, stop, and change the deeply rooted behaviors that are negatively impacting the survivor's relationships. Friends and family should be understanding and forgiving as the survivor recovers at his own pace.

Chapter 14

Effects of Childhood Trauma through the Lifespan

Cris Ann Scaglione. Ph.D.
The Chicago School of Professional Psychology

Childhood trauma has many "trickle-up" effects throughout the lifespan. The shocking violations of trust, security, and boundaries caused by trauma, abuse or neglect, as well as the associated experiences of profound psychological and/or physical pain, deeply affect psychological and physical well-being. This is especially true in childhood, when we are less physically, cognitively, socially, and emotionally prepared to understand and cope with trauma. Children are developmentally vulnerable and in need of care and guided age-appropriate challenges that promote their development into happy, healthy, functioning adults. This prolonged period of development (nearly two decades) is necessary for our tremendous intellectual and social/cultural growth. Disrupting its trajectory has numerous long-term effects.

Children (especially when traumatized before their sense of identity and verbal skills are developed) have great difficulty understanding trauma, how to express it, and how to begin integrating it into the story of their lives and the many facets of their selfhood. This does not mean that considerable resilience and life skills are not developed by many, if not most, children exposed to trauma, abuse or neglect. However, it is inevitable that childhood trauma will influence their development as people, leaving them with challenges that might be different, more numerous and/or more intense than those that confront the non-traumatized.

Trauma overwhelms the ability to cope with a situation. It unseats our mental and physical equilibrium. Maintaining homeostasis is the main function of much of our brain, as well as our endocrine and immune systems. Disrupting this balance is the primary avenue by which trauma affects our mental and physical health. Too often, the many forms of abuse that can be visited upon a child are also repeated, creating chronic or "complex" trauma. In general, the more severe and repeated the trauma, and the younger the age at which it started, the more indelible and widespread its effects.

The aftermath of childhood trauma clearly highlights body-mind interactions. Much of what is known about the effects of childhood trauma focuses on problems with mental and emotional health. However, physical health is also at risk as the ACES, the Adverse Childhood Events Study by the Centers for Disease Control and Prevention (CDC) and Kaiser Permanente, has shown (Dong, et al., 2005). Disruption of the normal pace, stages and challenges of development often impedes the ability of a child or teenager to make social connections and develop a solid sense of self, let alone self-esteem and a realistic sense of worth and competence. Often, attention, academic skills, and behavioral or emotional control can be impaired, possibly resulting in "acting out," aggression, and bullying. Social isolation, anxiety, depression, and frank post-traumatic stress disorder (PTSD) are also common.

In adulthood, disorders such as depression, anxiety, PTSD, and dissociative and personality disorders are associated with childhood abuse. Addictions, eating disorders, suicidal thinking and non-suicidal self-injury are also common. Like many symptoms of mental distress, many of these problems are attempts to resolve, alleviate, or numb the intense, confusing, and overwhelmingly negative feelings and thoughts that can result from trauma. Even without a fully diagnosable disorder, it is common to struggle with sadness, fear, doubt, insecurity, intrusive negative thoughts and memories, distrust, nightmares, and mood swings. Goal-directed action, attention, problem-solving, follow-through, maintaining a coherent sense of self, and appropriate emotional control can also be problematic.

Trauma can also affect physical health, independently of any physical injuries that may have occurred during childhood abuse or neglect. Trauma, especially complex trauma, can weaken the immune system, making people more susceptible to illnesses. It can also trigger auto-immune conditions like rheumatoid arthritis and fibromyalgia (Boscarino, 2004; Stojanovich &

Marisavljevich, 2008). Childhood trauma has also been implicated in some neurological conditions like Alzheimer's disease (Burri, Maercker, Krammer & Simmen-Janevska, 2013).

A well-documented result of traumatic experience is that the brain systems involved with emotional regulation, appropriate decision-making, and self-control — the frontal-subcortical circuits — can be disrupted (Karl, Schaefer, Malta, Dörfel, Rohleder & Werner, 2006; Koenen et al., 2001; Leskin & White, 2007; Weber & Reynolds, 2004). Early childhood trauma can also impair and distort the development of the right hemisphere of the brain, making it difficult to accurately read social cues and interpret and express emotion for the entirety of the person's life. This phenomenon is rooted in Bowlby's attachment theory, and has been well documented by Schore (e.g. 2000), whose work initiated a new interdisciplinary field known as "interpersonal neurobiology."

The turmoil of traumatized people may be most evident in their relationships. Most childhood trauma is relational — a person important to the child's well-being was abusive, or "lost" through injury, death, or illness (physical or mental). With chronic and complex trauma, it was often many people who were abusive or unavailable. In the process of recovering from trauma, children (and adults) are often re-traumatized, often by others in a position of power or authority, who do not believe or understand what happened, or are insensitive in their reactions. These events almost guarantee that children exposed to trauma will have ongoing negative expectations of people and relationships.

The desire for stability, safety, meaningful connection, and intimacy in our relationships with others is one of the most basic and powerful of human motivations—indeed it is necessary to our survival as individuals and as a species. Yet experiences of intense fear, disgust, anger, and grief associated with relationships understandably create profound barriers to even some of the simple interpersonal connections. Traumatized men can be especially ill-equipped to deal with this, since they are usually not socialized to be emotionally expressive, candid, and vulnerable in relationships. An argument can be made that men's socialization is in and of itself traumatizing at times. At the very least, it does not improve their chances of healing relational wounds, especially ones founded in childhood abuse.

Instead, both men and women who have endured childhood trauma can develop bad habits when interacting with others or defending themselves against connection with others. The combination of changes to the brain and personal psychology that occur from trauma results in traumatized adults being hypersensitive to signs of possible danger, often withdrawing, and being quick to feel a blend of intense negative emotions—shame, unworthiness, anger, terror, distrust etc. Approach-avoidance patterns, which must be negotiated in any relationship, are even more challenging for adults traumatized as children, especially during conflict. Unfortunately, it is also possible to bring abusive patterns of thought and action, modeled by childhood abuser(s), into adult relationships. As much as the experiences of childhood trauma and abuse were reviled, they will nonetheless form at least part of the template for future interpersonal relationships.

One of the most adaptive responses to trauma is to seek support and assistance from others, including peers, professionals, and fellow survivors. Yet this may be one of the most difficult things to attempt since interpersonal injury is at the core of most childhood trauma. Nonetheless, meaningful connections with trustworthy, empathetic people go a long way to repair trauma and allow interrupted developmental processes to unfold. Recovery works best when people understand that the process takes a long time (probably lifelong) and that trauma is complex. Many sources of support and intervention are likely to be needed. It is also important for traumatized adults and their friends and family to accept without harshness the myriad lingering effects of trauma, and to be patient with the process. As with most recovery it is also crucial to remember that you are not alone, and when you can, reach out to receive or provide assistance.

References

Boscarino, J. A. (2004). Posttraumatic stress disorder and physical illness: results from clinical and epidemiologic studies. *Annals of the New York Academy of Sciences, 1032*(1), 141-153.

Burri, A., Maercker, A., Krammer, S., & Simmen-Janevska, K. (2013). Childhood trauma and PTSD symptoms increase the risk of cognitive impairment in a sample of former indentured child laborers in old age. *PLoS ONE, 8*(2), e57826. http://doi.org/10.1371/journal.pone.0057826

Dong, M., Anda, R. F., Felitti, V. J., Williamson, D. F., Dube, S. R., Brown, D. W., & Giles, W. H. (2005). Childhood residential mobility and multiple health risks during adolescence and adulthood: the hidden role of adverse childhood experiences. *Archives of Pediatrics & Adolescent Medicine, 159*(12), 1104-1110.

Karl, A., Schaefer, M., Malta, L. S., Dörfel, D., Rohleder, N., & Werner, A. (2006). A meta-analysis of structural brain abnormalities in PTSD. *Neuroscience & Biobehavioral Reviews, 30*(7), 1004-1031

Koenen, K. C., Driver, K. L., Oscar-Berman, M., Wolfe, J., Folsom, S., Huang, M. T., & Schlesinger, L. (2001). Measures of prefrontal system dysfunction in posttraumatic stress disorder. *Brain & Cognition, 45*, 64-78.

Leskin, L. P. & White, P. M. (2007). Attentional networks reveal executive function deficits in posttraumatic stress disorder. *Neuropsychology, 21,* 275-284.

Liberzon, I. & Sripada C. S. (2008). The functional neuroanatomy of PTSD: A critical review. *Progress in Brain Research, 167,* 151–169.

Schore A. N. (2000). Attachment and the regulation of the right brain. *Attachment and Human Development, 2*(1), 23-47.

Stojanovich, L., & Marisavljevich, D. (2008). Stress as a trigger of autoimmune disease. *Autoimmunity Reviews, 7*(3), 209-213.

Weber, D. A., & Reynolds, C. R. (2004). Clinical perspectives on neurobiological effects of psychological trauma. *Neuropsychology Review, 14*(2), 115-129.

Chapter 15 Summary

Male Abuse Survivors and Relationships

Dr. Raymond Nourmand describes abuse as the experience of "being in a situation against one's will, where feelings of angst or pain are experienced." Abuse can be an event, or a state of being – lasting for days, weeks, months, or even years.

Abuse manifests through a survivor's life in many ways. (See the chapter titled "Manifestations of Trauma.") Dr. Nourmand explains in detail how abuse challenges and reshapes our perception of the world. It no longer becomes a safe place.

Recovery from experiences of abuse is contingent on several factors. Personality, level of functioning before the abuse, and social support, among other factors that are discussed in detail in the following chapter, determine what the recovery process will look like.

Dr. Nourmand stresses that the core of recovery is communication. Talking about the abuse with someone relieves much of the feelings of guilt and shame burdening nearly all survivors of sexual abuse. He goes on to discuss how humans are built to communicate and relate to one another, and that by doing so, survivors create much needed social support systems.

Men traditionally have been put into a "man-box" where they are told they need to "suck it up" or "man up" when faced with adversity. This ideology is errant from our natural needs and desires as human beings to express how we are feeling. Additionally, this traps men in a dilemma where they face being looked at as "less of a man" for speaking out or having to deal with the trauma alone.

Issues of intimacy and vulnerability are hallmarks for male survivors, as Dr. Nourmand explains, but these issues can be worked through and recovery is possible.

For me, as a spouse, and what Dr. Nourmand echoes in the following chapter, it is important to identify that education is the first step in understanding and recovery. It took me 12 years to realize that Robert's behavior had nothing to do with me. It stemmed from his abuse, which happened long before I was in his life. When I get into a dark place, I have to remind myself that I am neither the cause nor the cure. Then I need to be grateful for what I do have: a great husband and a wonderful father.

I'm not a survivor and I can never adequately understand what that is like. But I can arm myself with education. I seek to understand my husband and male survivors. The more I learn, the less I internalize.

Chapter 15

Male Abuse Survivors and Relationships

By Raymond Nourmand, Ph.D.
American Jewish University

Often when we hear or see the word "abuse," we think of intense physical, sexual, or emotional violations. After all, when the word "abuse" comes up, that is what most people are usually referring to. However, when we look at it from a different perspective, abuse can be more broadly understood as the experience of being in any situation against one's own will, where one feels intense pain and anguish at the hands of another, with no perceived escape route for a critical period of time. This could be for seconds, hours, days, weeks, months, or even years.

Whenever a person experiences any kind of abuse, there is a reasonable chance that he or she is going to experience some kind of mental, emotional, and or even physical backlash. By nature, abuse is almost always an intense, unpredictable, and overwhelming experience to the person on the receiving side. Being on the receiving side of abuse normally challenges a person's sense of personal safety, order, and control in the world. As humans, we like to think that the world is an orderly place, where things are always under control, and that, consequently, nothing very unpleasant will happen to us. We like to think that the world is safe, sound, and trustworthy. While we may intellectually grasp that unpleasant things may happen to us because we see them happening to others, it is reasonable to suspect that no one naturally expects unpleasant things to happen to him or her personally. Maybe this is a defense to help us go through our day more comfortably, a way to reduce our fear and worry of what can -possibly happen, a way to make us feel safe and secure in a world that at times seems chaotic. Yet, when abuse happens, often these beliefs get immediately challenged. All of a sudden, the world no longer seems to be the safe, predictable, pleasant place we envisioned it to be. It is not as secure, orderly, and trustworthy as we would have liked to believe. As such, survivors are almost always confronted with a very real sense of fear, vulnerability, and being out-of-control that can take weeks, months, years, or even a lifetime to understand and come to terms with.

The extent to which a person will successfully recover from his or her experience with abuse is likely related to various factors. For example, it is important to look at the subjective intensity of the abuse, the survivor's level of functioning before the abuse took place, the way he or she tended to cope with adversity before the abuse, personality characteristics, and perceived social support. Generally, the less intense the abuse, the better the person's functioning pre-abuse, the more hardy and resilient the person pre-abuse, and the greater the perceived social support, the better the prognosis seems to be. In other words, it is important to look at the answers to the following questions: How did the survivor experience the abuse? How equipped was he or she to deal with this kind of abuse effectively? Had he or she been through similar hardships before? If so, how did he or she cope with them? Does he or she feel adequately supported or cared for socially?

At the crux of any successful survivorship, it seems key that the survivor become comfortable talking about what happened, about how he or she felt, and about any residual effects the abuse has had on him or her in an open and honest manner. This kind of communication can be helpful in addressing feelings like loneliness, shame, and guilt, which tend to be common among survivors. The loss of control that often accompanies abuse almost always carries with it a feeling of being alone, isolated, and that "no one will ever understand what I am talking about or what I have been through." It is painful. Shame and guilt often come in to play as coping mechanisms to help the survivor deal with the uncontrollability of the abuse. It seems as though that as long as someone feels intense and persistent shame and guilt over the abuse, the more he or she is trying to assume responsibility for what happened. The underlying thought pattern is, "I must have done something wrong to get this; I need to be more careful next time." At the core of these feelings is the desire to gain control, ostensibly a direct reaction to feeling so out of control during the abuse.

Sharing about these feelings and others can be a big step in the right direction.

Communication can be viewed as a fundamental aspect of creating a sense of support and connection. As humans, we are wired to relate and connect with one another. We express ourselves to one another because doing so allows us to feel like we belong, we matter, that our story is both unique and universal at the same time. Talking, writing, and other forms of expression allow other people to come into our world, and take a peek into how life looks from our personal perspective. It is very gratifying to feel understood. Nevertheless, if people persistently do not understand what we are going through, it is very easy for us to internalize this in such a vulnerable state, and feel like we do not have a place to belong in this world anymore. Yet, while talking about, writing about, or otherwise communicating our true inner experiences can be helpful in reducing loneliness, shame, guilt, and foster a sense of connection and belonging, sometimes getting to this point of directly expressing what is really going inside can be a real challenge, especially for survivors who are male.

From the beginning of time, society has told men that when experiencing stress, adversity, and calamity, they need to "be strong." They need to hide what they are feeling inside. They need to "suck it up." They should "keep a stiff upper lip," and "take it like a man." In sum, our culture persistently discourages men from showing, let alone talking about, their true inner thoughts and feelings.

When people feel sad, angry, hurt, scared, worried and other unpleasant feelings, our bodies are naturally wired to express those emotions and release that energy. Our emotions are there for a reason. They are meant to be there. They are signals. They are our bodies' ways of telling us that something is going on, something needs attention, something needs to be addressed. To disrupt that natural process can be really damaging to one's overall health. Indeed, studies have shown that when people suppress their unpleasant emotions, they are more likely to report feeling stressed than those who do express their discomfort.

While women have traditionally been socialized to express themselves, for some reason the opposite message has been passed down to men. Somewhere, somehow, along the development of society, men have been repeatedly told to avoid expressing their feelings, discouraged from talking about what is going on inside them, and told that to share their feelings is "bad," "wrong," and that they should effectively "stop it." This socially imposed double-standard on expressing one's self likely complicates the way males experience abuse altogether. By being socialized to not talk about their true experiences, male survivors are often faced with a dilemma: stay quiet to fit in, or speak up at the risk of getting labeled as "broken," "defective," or "weak."

Consequently, male survivors are likely to be in an especially tough spot when it comes to intimate relationships. The very tools that are required to make intimate relationships flourish are the very things that male survivors are likely to struggle with more-so than others: namely, the willingness to be open, honest, and vulnerable. For any human being, being open, honest, and vulnerable is usually a challenge. Any time we open ourselves up to somebody, we are in some way submitting to him or her, risking the possibility of being rejected by him or her. And indeed, the more personal the level of self-disclosure is, the more powerful this potential rejection becomes, and thus the scarier the overall experience can be. Accordingly, when one considers the idea that survivors of abuse are probably more sensitive to feeling out of control than those who have not experienced such abuse, the idea of willfully making oneself vulnerable can become a more complicated endeavor. After all, the survivor is likely to deep down think to him or herself, "The last time I was out of control I was devastated. I was hurt, pained, and taken advantage of in ways I never want to experience again. I don't want to go through that again. It hurt too much." Being out of control, which is required when making oneself vulnerable, is probably something male survivors are skeptical about and wary of, at least in the beginning. Add to this the pressure of being a male member of society, effectively being told that to open up is a sign of weakness, and the issue just keeps getting more complicated.

However, there is good news. While male survivors of abuse might have an especially difficult time opening up and being willfully vulnerable for the reasons mentioned above, they can also be remarkably resilient. This is precisely one of the main purposes of this book: to share the message that there is hope, and that things can get better!

An important key to helping male survivors flourish in their relationships is to understand that they have special needs that they may or may not initially feel comfortable expressing. First, male survivors are likely to be particularly sensitive to making themselves vulnerable given how abuse tends to affect people. The nature of abuse is such that the survivor is often left feeling a remarkable sense of fear, mistrust, and being out of control immediately after the abuse has begun, and probably for some time afterwards. Of course, there is considerable variation within different survivors as to what extent they are likely to feel such pain and for how long. At the same time, however, it is reasonable to suspect that such intense experiences are likely to leave survivors feeling extra cautious about becoming out of control again, which is what strong, intimate relationships generally require – stepping into the unknown and making oneself vulnerable. Second, male survivors are likely to be hesitant to opening up about their experiences due to social pressures that dictate if men express any sense of vulnerability, they are weak, defective, and "less manly." This can make it especially challenging for a man to be truly vulnerable, as he is likely wary of being criticized and ostracized for sharing his truth when it does not fit traditional male stereotypes of being "strong," "powerful," and "in control" at all times. Finally, male survivors are likely to need extra care and patience at least in the immediate aftermath of their first disclosures of their experience with abuse. It is very important that when a male survivor takes that first risk of opening himself up, he is listened to caringly, sensitively, and patiently. It is important to be accepting of his experience, and to communicate to him that he is still loved, accepted, and cherished despite what he has gone through. He is not broken. He is not crazy. He is not weak. He is brave. He is courageous. He is strong. For talking about it.

Being mindful of what abuse is, how it affects people, and the unique challenges that male survivors experience can be very beneficial for those who have close relationships with male survivors of abuse. It may sound clichéd but education is a vital first step. The more a person can understand where a survivor is coming from, and translate that understanding into open, honest, and sensitive action, the more he or she is setting him or herself up for the potential of a truly wonderful relationship. Moreover, it is important to keep in mind that we all come from our own backgrounds, with our own unique stories, with our own challenges and struggles as individuals. The reality is that the more we come to understand ourselves, and appreciate how we have been affected by people in our own lives, the more we can truly understand other people and really be there for them. The truth is: the more we understand ourselves, the more we can accurately understand others. The more we get in touch with our own experiences of pain, hurt, frustrations, worries, anxieties, and disappointments, the more likely we are to truly understand and sensitively interact with those who might be struggling with these feelings in their own ways.

Furthermore, education about abuse, knowledge of social pressures, and personal awareness appear to be at the heart of building great relationships with people who are male survivors. As members of society, as family members, as partners, the more we come to see that their pain is not just their pain, but also our pain, the more likely we are to act in ways that will convey to them that they are not alone, that they do matter, and that they are still lovable.

Chapter 16 Summary

Psychopharmacological Approaches to Trauma Treatment

For the purpose of this chapter, Dr. Richard Sinacola defines trauma as, "an obstacle that is, for a time, insurmountable by the use of customary methods of problem solving...an upset in the steady state of the individual" (Caplan, 1961). This definition is congruent and compatible with other definitions used in this book, specifically the working definition I use in the chapter titled "My Husband's Abuse," and the definition that Dr. Nourmand uses in his chapter, "Understanding Male Survivors." As noted in the following chapter, trauma is unique to the individual, and is based on his or her perceptions of an event. Two people, from different backgrounds, experiencing different life events, may perceive the same situation totally differently. One may feel that they have been abused and as a result are traumatized, while the other may not.

If an individual perceives the event as traumatic, it will likely result in emotional distress and impair the ability of the individual to function. How people perceive and deal with trauma is based on several factors. Sinacola states that life experiences, IQ, and even our financial resources all factor into how we perceive, and subsequently treat, our trauma. Obviously, those who are situated well financially have more resources to use on treatment. However, all the money in the world is of no use if the survivor does not want to deal with their trauma. Many survivors (including Robert for a long time) want to shut that door and never look behind it again.

Sinacola emphasizes that the pharmacological approach is not meant to be the sole source of treatment, but rather to be used in conjunction with other treatment tools such as psychotherapy. Sinacola stresses the importance of psychotherapy in trauma survivors, especially within the first few days of the abuse.

Sinacola also discusses the importance of the "medical home," which he describes as the co-operation and communication between all of the specialists providing care to the patient. This medical home starts with the primary care physician and includes therapists, psychiatrists, and any other specialists that are needed to treat the survivor.

The general consensus is that there is no single medicinal solution for PTSD. Rather, medications should be used to treat the varying symptoms that may arise from trauma.

One of the common symptoms of PTSD is sleeplessness. Sinacola presents the effects and benefits of several different kinds of medication used to treat this symptom. He does the same with medications used to treat the other common symptoms of PTSD such as mood disorders, anxiety, paranoid thoughts, and more.

Sinacola emphasizes that it is crucial for care providers to be aware of past substance abuse histories of patients. Substance abuse is a common manifestation of trauma, and a significant portion of male survivors seeking care will have a history of it. There are alternative, non-narcotic medications and treatment plans for survivors who have a history of substance abuse.

Throughout Robert's youth and into his first marriage, he used substances as a coping mechanism. He has since stopped using any substances to cope. He now uses proper medication that helps with his mood and reduces the symptoms that arise from his abuse.

Communication and trust is key when working with survivors. There has to be good working relationships between caregivers and the survivor, as well as communication between all professionals who are providing care. This ensures a stronger, holistic, more effective recovery.

Chapter 16

Psychopharmacological Approaches to Trauma Treatment

Richard S. Sinacola, Ph.D.
Licensed Psychologist and Consultant, Pasadena, CA

Adjunct Professor MFT Program,
The Chicago School of Professional Psychology

Lecturer in Psychology and Education,
California State University–Los Angeles

When one stops to think about all the potential sources of trauma and crisis an individual is exposed to on a daily basis, it is no surprise to realize that in the course of one's life there is most likely going to be an event that leads to a person needing counseling or medication to deal with the chaos caused by exposure to a traumatic event. While individuals may define their personal trauma or crisis in their own terms, the definition that works for the purposes of this chapter best describes trauma as, "an obstacle that is, for a time, insurmountable by the use of customary methods of problem solving...an upset in the steady state of the individual," (Caplan, 1961). Here we see that it is the experience of trauma or crisis and the individual's unique perception of it that determine the nature of the effect, if any, on the individual and his/her ability to function. In fact, trauma usually has four parts (Kanel, 2015):

1. A precipitating event occurs.
2. The person has a perception of the event as threatening or damaging.
3. This perception leads to emotional distress.
4. The distress leads to impairment in functioning due to a failure of the usual coping mechanisms.

If the individual does not perceive the event as traumatic or necessarily noteworthy, then they will not be affected by it and the third and fourth steps or parts would not be cause for concern. Kanel (2015) points out that there are certain personality traits or particulars that seem to indicate when a person may be more resilient or when they may be more at risk for being affected by trauma. Persons who are older tend to be bothered less by traumatic events. Perhaps their life experiences have caused an "inoculation" effect on future crisis situations. Persons who are well traveled and who have had numerous life experiences such as serving in the military, working as a missionary in a foreign land, or working in the Peace Corp tend to be more resilient. Individuals with higher IQs tend to be able to reason some of their stress and trauma away when compared to those with lower IQs. Not surprisingly, those with greater financial resources tend to weather trauma better. They appear to have the means to hire good attorneys, physicians, and other professionals when they need then, and they have the means to "buy" what they need to improve the situation. Additionally, the field of ego psychology reminds us that persons identified to have good "ego strengths" tend to cope better when they experience a crisis or trauma. Typically good ego strengths include the ability to be flexible and adaptive, tolerant, and optimistic. Finally, people with a history of mental illness such as depression, bipolar illness, anxiety, and psychotic spectrum illness tend not to do as well then they experience crisis and trauma, and these events are likely to trigger a bout of mental illness when they are experienced by the individual. (Kanel, 2015).

What we consider the sources of trauma and crisis: natural disasters, acts of violence and terrorism, sexual assault, domestic violence, serious or life-threatening illness, death of a loved one, loss of income, or repeated exposure to violent or unpleasant situations in which the individual has little control. It is clear that there are many situations and events which could cause or trigger a crisis in the individual. For many who succumb to the chaos and manifest symptoms, we see a variety of anxiety and mood spectrum disorders. Some of the more common disorders include various adjustment disorders such as Adjustment Disorder with Anxious Mood, Depressed Mood or both; PTSD and Acute Stress Disorder; Anxiety Disorder NOS and Depressive Disorder NOS. There is also exacerbations of already existing mood or psychotic spectrum illnesses like Major Depressive Illness; Borderline Personality

Disorder, Generalized Anxiety Disorder, OCD, Schizophrenia, and Bipolar Illness. When this occurs, it is imperative that assistance be provided quickly to normalize the event and prevent the need for a major hospitalization. The actual biological etiology of PTSD and other trauma related conditions is beyond the scope of this chapter, but research has demonstrated that prolonged exposure to stress changes the function and structure of the nervous system; namely, the hypothalamic-pituitary-adrenal axis that may in fact lead to a dysregulation of our *fight/flight* system resulting in impairment (Raison & Miller, 2003).

While the goals of psychotherapy vary from one school of thought to another, it is widely known that intervention should ideally be provided within days of the event or trauma to prevent lasting traumatic perceptions or memories from taking hold (Kanel, 2015). Clinicians typically follow an A-B-C model which involves: A. *Achieving* rapport with the client by providing Appropriate Attending behaviors; B. *Boiling* the issue down and getting to the Basics of the problem; C. Re-establishing and assessing the patient's *Coping* skills (Jones, 1968). Therapy should attempt to establish rapport quickly and assist the patient with changing his or her perception of the event where possible. Taking adequate history assists the therapist with the facts and exactly how the patient perceives the problem and the intensity of the effect. All therapists need to understand what types of coping skills the patient has used in the past and if they have been effective. In most cases the approach is threefold – it consists of therapy or counseling, providing resources, and providing medication as needed. (Sinacola, 2015).

Here, the clinician provides counseling or psychotherapy in an individual or group format utilizing various evidenced-based treatments. Psychoanalytic, existential, CBT, and REBT have all been evaluated in the treatment of those with trauma issues. Mindfulness techniques, hypnosis, and EMDR have all been shown to improve the situation for victims of trauma and crisis (Kanel, 2015; Shapiro & Forrest, 1997). For many patients experiencing crisis and trauma, the event itself generates the need for other services or information. Often the patient needs to obtain legal counsel for issues related to the event or the individual needs an expert medical evaluation. These resources may be nothing more than a referral to another professional or they may take the form of disseminating information about self-help groups or classes in the area. In some cases, bibliotherapy is suggested with a list of books or videos to view or discuss.

Finally, medication may need to be utilized to assist the patient in optimal functioning or to prevent the situation from worsening. Most experts agree that there is no one best medication for PTSD or trauma survivors and that medications should be used to address a cluster of related symptoms (Briere & Scott, 2006). When considering if a medication consultation may be needed, consider the following:

1. Have the patient's symptoms worsened in the last several weeks?

2. Is the patient unable to sleep, eat, or work?
3. Is he or she feeling suicidal or hopeless?
4. Does the patient have a history of a mood disorder?
5. Does the patient have a substance abuse history? If so, inform the prescriber.

Many licensed therapists forget that failure to refer a patient for a medication consultation (when their situation or condition would suggest that they would benefit from one) is, in and of itself, grounds for malpractice. When considering the questions mentioned above, it would be wise to assess the patient each week they are in treatment with you, and if you notice that their symptoms are not improving, then begin a dialogue with them about medication. It is important to emphasize that medication is simply a tool, part of the treatment plan, and in no way diminishes the role or importance of talk therapy. For many patients with past episodes of major depression or psychotic manifestations, it is important to intervene early to prevent a more serious episode or break-down. Certainly, if a patient is unable to sleep and is getting increasingly more agitated during the day because of this, it is not necessary to have the patient suffer needlessly. Sleep aides, sedating antidepressants, or sedative-hypnotics could be utilized with an awareness of the patient's personal substance use history. One must make sure that he or she is not given any medication that could be abused if they have a history of doing this.

One of the more disruptive symptoms for patients who have experienced a trauma is agitation and sleeplessness. There are three types of insomnia typical to patients with mental illness or trauma situations: initial insomnia or the inability to relax and fall asleep; middle insomnia or the ability to fall asleep followed by periodic bouts of awakening throughout the night resulting in exhaustion in the morning; and finally, terminal insomnia where the patient falls asleep just fine but awakens at about three or four in the morning unable to return to sleep with complaints of daytime sleepiness (Sinacola & Peters-Strickland, 2012).

Research has shown that patients who typically experience initial insomnia are more likely to be experiencing anxiety or a crisis situation. Patients with no history of sleep issues who have begun to experience middle insomnia are also plagued with stress or most likely dealing with a crisis. While chronic stress has been known to decrease amounts of serotonin in the central nervous system, chronic depression and the presence of a mood disorder has been known to contribute to terminal and middle insomnia, as well. Assuming adequate history information has been taken, and one is reasonably sure that the patient does not have a history of substance abuse, there are several options for improving sleep and reducing agitation at bedtime.

Patients need to be educated that using over the counter sleep aids or alcohol may add to the problem in the future and cause increased amounts of depression over time. For patients who have experienced a recent traumatic event and who present with the inability to relax at bedtime and sleep, an appropriate sleep medication may be suggested. Benzodiazepine receptor agonists like Ambien (zolpidem), Lunesta (eszopiclone), and Sonata (zaleplon) are designed to act quickly and assist with initial and middle insomnia. Taken as directed for a short period of time (2-3 weeks) these are effective in restoring sleep so a patient can continue to function. A newer medication known as an orexin antagonist is available, as well. Belsomra (suvorexant) works to calm these active neurotransmitters in the CNS. Keep in mind that all of these substances have been known to become habit forming when taken in larger amounts and for longer periods then initially anticipated.

If your patient has a history of alcohol or substance abuse, it is best to avoid using benzodiazepines such as Xanax (alprazolam), Ativan (lorazepam), or Klonopin (clonazepam) to control anxiety and/or to induce sleep. Exceptions are made if panic disorder has been confirmed and diagnosed. It is not a good idea to consider barbiturates for controlling agitation and managing sleep. These are extremely habit forming and may lead to unintentional overdoses. Furthermore, some believe that the use of benzodiazepines may in fact interfere with the psychological processing of traumatic memories (Briere & Scott, 2006). There is essentially only one non-habit forming sleep formulation known as Rozerem (ramelteon). It is designed to work with your natural levels of melatonin acting as a melatonin receptor agonist.

For patients with substance abuse issues the use of sedating antidepressants offer the best options. These medications increase serotonin and naturally improve sleep over time. They also have the added benefit of improving mood and reducing obsessive tendencies often seen in those who have had a recent trauma situation. Some suggest that SSRIs may in fact improve both the function and physical structure of various neurological structures needed for healthy emotion (Briere & Scott, 2006). These medications include most of the SSRIs such as Prozac (fluoxetine), Zoloft (sertraline), Paxil (paroxetine), Celexa (citalopram) and Lexapro (esitalopram), as well as the SNRI Effexor (venlafaxine). There are newer SSRIs and SPARIs available. These include Brintellix and Viibryd, but to date, they only have approval for use in patients with depression. Some of the older tricyclic medications like amitriptyline and doxepin are very sedating, but watch for several of the other anticholinergic side effects like dizziness, dry mouth, constipation, blurred vision, and orthostatic hypotension. Newer generation serotonin-5HT2 receptor antagonists like trazodone and nefazodone are sedating and less likely to cause as many anticholinergic issues. The heterocyclic medication Remeron (mirtazepine) is rather sedating, but watch for an increase in weight and appetite especially at lower doses.

There has been an increase in physicians and other prescribers using very sedating antipsychotic medications to assist agitated patients who report insomnia. Unless the patient is psychotic, seriously agitated, or a danger to himself or others, these medications should not be routinely used to induce sleep or control anxiety. Most if these medications carry serious side effect profiles and can cause changes in one's weight, cholesterol profiles, and metabolism. These are also not a good idea for the elderly or cardiac patients as many of these have been known to cause potentially fatal cardiac arrhythmias that could lead to a stroke. One medication in particular, Seroquel (quetiapine), is very sedating and is sometimes used as an alternative sleep aid. This should not be considered unless others have failed and the patient has psychotic or bipolar manifestations. The side-effect profile is considerably higher than most sleep medications, even the benzodiazepines (Sinacola & Peters-Strickland, 2012).

Patients who were exposed to traumatic events who later have symptoms related to PTSD and acute stress disorder may need to consider medications that not only reduce mood issues and anxiety, but calm paranoid thinking, night terrors, and nighttime agitation. When paranoid or psychotic thinking is present, the use of atypical antipsychotics may be needed. Sedating medications are most helpful, especially if the patient cannot sleep or is agitated. While most of them will work to reduce symptoms, some like quetiapine and olanzepine are more sedating. Low-dose risperidone and aripiprasole help to reduce symptoms with less overall potential for both anticholinergic and extra pyramidal effects like potential harmful movement disorders (tardive dyskinesia) (Sinacola & Peters-Strickland, 2012). The use of mood stabilizers/anticonvulsants like Lamictal (lamotrigine), Depakote (valproate), and Topamax (topiramate) show promise in reducing mood swings and emotional agitation in patients exposed to trauma who complain of labile agitation. Some like Neurontin (gabapentin) are very sedating and may effectively be used before bedtime to assist with sleep. Many patients experience nightmares or night terrors as a result of their exposure and feel "re-traumatized" when they sleep as dreams remind them of the events. For these patients, the use of the adrenergic inhibiting agent Prazosin reduces these occurrences. Some research suggests that using propranolol soon after exposure to a traumatic event may interfere with how some of these memories are stored in the nervous system (Nugent et al., 2010). The use of alpha and beta-adrenergic agonists appears to be mainly for reducing hyperarousal and sleep disturbance.

Medications that are more noradrenergic or dopaminergic may be too excitatory for most patients with issues related to anxiety and trauma. Stimulating antidepressants should be avoided along with the use of actual stimulants like methyphenidate or amphetamine mixed salts, unless of course, the patient has already been tested and diagnosed with ADHD. Pain killers and analgesics should also be avoided due to their high risk for addiction. While analgesics and opioid-based medications reduce pain and cause a calming effect in an anxious person, they offer no redeeming pharmacologic benefits over time.

It is important for the mental health clinician to realize that he or she is part of a treatment team designed to assist the patient with getting better and maintaining his or her gains. Often times, the non-medical therapist feels ill equipped to discuss the need for a medication consultation with the very professionals who are providing them. In the health care milieu today, the "medical home" model radiates out from the patient's primary care provider (PCP) who coordinates care from several specialists and services. He or she should be consulted and the PCP will decide if they are comfortable with providing the medication in question or if a psychiatrist or clinical nurse specialist is needed. The therapist must feel comfortable initiating the referral and consulting with the prescriber to assure that the prescriber is aware of all symptoms and the scope of the presenting concern. The therapist is also the person who sees the patient on a weekly basis and can alert the prescriber to any side effects or reactions, as well as provide regular updates on patient progress. Prescribers typically appreciate timely feedback and do not expect non-medical providers to be well versed on the medications and their expectations. They do, however, appreciate some awareness of the diagnosis and the medications indicated for their treatment. If a particular prescriber is not responsive to therapist feedback and is essentially ignoring his or her input, another provider should be sought and the PCP informed of the need for another referral. It is important that all members of the "medical home" team work together in the service of the patient.

Remember that patients who have experienced trauma events are often scared and a bit distrusting of others. They are more likely to listen to or believe others who have experienced trauma than the professionals treating them. It is important to offer them guidance and companionate patience to facilitate the therapeutic alliance. Having a good working relationship over time will assure that the patient is engaged in the treatment process and likely to remain in treatment until the issues are resolved.

References

Briere, J., & Scott, C. (2006). Principles of trauma therapy: A guide to symptoms, evaluation, and treatment. Thousand Oaks, CA: Sage Publications.

Caplan, G. (1961). *An approach to community mental health.* New York: Grune & Stratton.

James, R., & Gilliland, B. (2013). *Crisis intervention strategies (7th Ed.).* Pacific Grove, CA: Brooks/Cole.

Janosik, E. (1986). *Crisis counseling: A contemporary approach.* Monterey, CA: Jones and Bartlett.

Jones, W. (1968). The ABC method of crisis management. *Mental Hygiene, 52,* 87-89.

Kanel, K. (2015). *A guide to crisis intervention (5th Ed.).* Stamford, CT: Cengage Learning.

Nugent, N., Christopher, N., Crow, J., Brown, L., Ostrowski, S., & Delahanty, D. (2010). The efficacy of early propranolol administration at reducing PTSD symptoms in pediatric injury patients: A pilot study. *Journal of Traumatic Stress, 23,* (2), 282-287.

Raison, C., & Miller, A. (2003). When enough is too much: The role of insufficient glucocorticoid signaling in the pathophysiology of stress related disorders. *American Journal of Psychiatry, 169,* 1554-1565.

Shapiro, F., & Forrest, M. (1997). *EMDR.* New York: Basic Books.

Sinacola, R. (2015, September). *The A-B-Cs of Trauma and Crisis Intervention.* Symposium presented at Pacific Oaks College – Pasadena, CA.

Sinacola, R., & Peters-Strickland, T. (2012). *Basic psychopharmacology for counselors and psychotherapists.* (2nd Ed.). Boston: Allyn and Bacon.

Chapter 17 Summary

Couples and Trauma:
Challenges and Opportunities

The only thing we have to bring to a relationship is our own experience, which is completely shaped by our past, as well as the values and norms that were imprinted upon us by our families and peer groups. As we grow, we acquire new experiences that help to shape and mold our perception of the world, like a piece of clay contoured by an artist – life. We rely on and draw from these experiences in our relationships with friends, family, spouses, and everyone else we come in contact with on a daily basis. While most of these daily interactions seem inconsequential and hold little importance, they are significant for two reasons – first, they add to the molding of our reality, and secondly, if they are negative or positive they will build on one another. The final straw doesn't break the camel's back; the weight of the straws underneath it does.

Our brains are much better at remembering negative experiences than positive ones; it's part of our psychology – the flight or fight response – and gave our caveman ancestors advantages that ensured the human species survived. The limbic system suited us well in alerting us to saber-toothed tigers and giant mastodons, but in 2017, those threats are in short supply, and the old warning systems can be detrimental to our interpersonal relationships.

Negative manifestations of this response are commonly found in male survivors, due to their post-traumatic stress from abuses suffered as children. These life experiences have molded their brains in such a way that they respond in a particular fashion to a threat – physical or mental. The top ways these stresses manifest in relationships is through avoidance and numbing.

Why doesn't he love me? and *He doesn't care about me,* are two frequent thoughts I had after a flare up with Robert. His avoidance of me and the problem at hand left me baffled and questioning his affection towards me. What I came to realize is that this was his way of trying to protect himself from what his mind told him was a threat. Male survivors want to distance themselves as much as they can from any source of conflict. This is true with Robert. Others will engage in risky behavior, including drugs and alcohol, to numb themselves.

The brain, as a malleable organ, can be changed and those old behaviors replaced by new ones. Therapy and positive experiences of working through issues in a healthy manner work to create healthier patterns in responses and relationships. They take time and effort, and the loving support of family and friends.

As spouses, we fall into our own roles within the relationship. A relationship with a male survivor will tend to lean towards imbalance. One person does more than the other, one is the caretaker or authority figure. There are many possible dynamics that can play out. In our relationship, I tend to do more and I make most of the decisions in the house. The finances, what car to buy, and other major household decisions are left up to me; I've accepted and embraced that role, and in doing so, the dynamic between us works.

I could write down a list of Robert's shortcomings - things that bother me or behaviors I wish he would or wouldn't do. I'm sure he could do the same for me as well! That is true for all of us in our relationships with others. What I have learned to do, and what takes true emotional growth, is to look inside myself at the things I can change, rather than hopelessly trying to change another person.

What I have described is a summary of what you will read in more detail in the following chapter, written by Dr. Melody Bacon, a specialist in the field of relationships and trauma. She describes the dynamic of couples and how trauma plays out in those relationships.

Chapter 17

Couples and Trauma:
Challenges and Opportunities

Melody Bacon, Ph.D.
The Chicago School of Professional Psychology

You can kiss your family and friends good-bye and put miles between you,
   but at the same time, you carry them with you in your heart, your mind, your stomach,
   because you do not just live in a world, but a world lives in you.
   ~Frederick Buechner

Human relationships are fraught with struggle, even in the best of circumstances. This is because people are complicated and complexity is magnified in marital relationships. Because marriage is a vulnerable relationship with divorce rates averaging around 50%, partners know that their marriage faces a probability of failure. This creates uncertainty and anxiety; add to this the impact of trauma, and it is easy to understand why marriages in which one partner has experienced trauma are particularly challenging.

This chapter will review the effect of trauma survival on couples within the context of typical marital challenges and dynamics. While the term "marriage" conveys various meanings, for our purposes marriage will be defined to include same-sex and heterosexual unions, as well as long-term common law relationships. Recognizing that each of these relationships has its unique set of challenges, it is still possible to speak of relational dynamics and patterns that are common to all such relationships.

Overview of Typical Marital Dynamics

Schnarch (2009) calls marriage a "people-growing machine." He argues that in every marriage, individuals will come to the end of what they know how to do to resolve conflict and eventually end up in emotional gridlock. This is when the true growth opportunity begins for each partner. This emotional gridlock usually occurs after a couple has been together about five to seven years, and, in fact, the 7-10 year point in a first marriage is a common time for divorce. As couples fail to resolve the impasse of gridlock, one or both decide they've married the wrong person, and file for divorce. Unfortunately, second marriages have a much higher divorce rate than first marriages: 75% according to some estimates. One reason for this is the added stressors of blended families, but it is also true that people often find themselves struggling with the same issues that they had in their first marriages. As the old saying goes "wherever you go, there you are." You are the constant in your life.

The Influence of the Family System

Part of what we consistently bring to our relationships are the skills, patterns and assumptions of our families of origin. One might say that "wherever you go, there *they* are." As poet and author, Fredrick Buechner points out, "you carry them with you in your heart, your mind, your stomach." Bowen Family Systems theory holds that individuals come into adulthood with certain defaults for regulating emotional intensity. These defaults, known as reactivity, while not innate, function in much the same way as an instinct in that they are generally unconscious, knee-jerk reactions. Thus an individual from a family that tends toward a high degree of emotional distance to regulate intensity and minimize conflict will bring this default into his or her adult relationships. When the emotional intensity increases in this person's marital relationship, he or she will move toward distancing as a means for lowering intensity and conflict. Conversely, those individuals whose families used emotional fusion as a way to regulate conflict will push for higher levels of togetherness. When emotional intensity increases, these individuals tend to insist on agreement at all costs and see disagreement as a sign of betrayal.

What this underscores is that humans are largely formed by experiences that become stored in the brain creating unique neuropathways. This means that during the most crucial years of development, our brains are formed within the context of our families of origin. How our families handled conflict has a significant impact on the skill sets we bring into our marriages later in life. We default to ingrained reactions whenever an event replicates something in our past. For example, if you are having conflict with your spouse, your brain will resort to old reactions formed throughout your childhood and usually formed by your family system long before you were born. Given this, making changes within the context of the family of origin offers the best chance for lasting change.

When this normal reactivity is overlaid with the experience of trauma, however, the ability to make such changes is compromised. This is because our brains are hardwired to hold onto negative experiences, particularly those that threaten survival. As Hanson (2013) explains, experiences matter, "not just for how they feel in the moment but for the lasting traces they leave in your brain," (p. 11). This means that threatening experiences are far more likely to leave an imprint than good experiences. This has to do with the way in which the brain binds memory with emotion in what Hanson (2013) describes as a built-in negativity bias so that painful, negative experiences have far more effect than enjoyable, positive experiences. This process takes place in the limbic (fight, flight, or freeze) system of the brain, particularly in the amygdale, which intertwines memory with its affective experience. Over time, one's amygdale becomes hypersensitive to negative experiences so that even relatively non-threatening experiences set off alarm bells and the survival mechanisms inherent in the brain release stress hormones like adrenaline, cortisol and norepinephrine. The cortisol overstimulates the brain and eventually will cause the hippocampus to shrink, making it even more difficult to soothe oneself and discern what is an actual threat (Hanson, 2013, p. 23).

But not all negative experiences are equal in intensity and, in fact, most are eventually stored as memories with increasingly lower levels of emotional and sensational intensity (van der Kolk and McFarlane, 1996). However, some events are so threatening and laden with emotional intensity that an individual is not able to process them effectively, setting the stage for developing PTSD. "Thus, paradoxically, the ability to transform memory is the norm," van der Kolk and McFarlane explain, "whereas in PTSD the full brunt of an experience does not fade with time" (p. 9).

The Impact of Trauma on Relationships

While PTSD is a multi-faceted diagnosis, there are certain issues associated with this diagnosis that directly affect an ability to form and maintain healthy relationships; these include: a tendency toward numbing of responsiveness, an inability to modulate physiological responses to stress, problems with distraction and stimulus discrimination and alterations in their psychological defense mechanisms and personal identity (van der Kolk and McFarlane, 1996, p. 9).

These issues have a direct correlation with how an individual is likely to react to normal marital stressors. For instance, avoidance and numbing will result in emotional distancing while chronic hyperarousal will manifest itself as a tendency to impulsively react to perceived threats. As van der Kolk and McFarlane (1996) explain, "The PTSD sufferers' inability to decipher messages from the autonomic nervous system interferes with their capacity to articulate how they are feeling (alexithymia) and makes them tend to react to their environment with either exaggerated or inhibited behaviors," (p. 13-14). "In adults," they elaborate, "it is expressed in impulsive behavior, excessive dependence, and a loss of capacity to make thoughtful, autonomous decisions," (p. 14).

This is particularly true of individuals who come from low-functioning families of origin which are characterized by high levels of emotional intensity resulting in neglect and abuse. Studies conducted by van der Kolk (1996) reveal that "traumatized adults with childhood histories of severe neglect have a particularly poor long-term prognosis as compared with traumatized individuals who had more secure attachment bonds as children" (p. 185). This would be in keeping with assumptions made by family systems theories that the emotional intensity of the family of origin affects the way in which adults manage relationships. It stands to reason that individuals who come into adulthood with deficits in self-soothing and emotional regulation would have difficulties in managing intimate relationships. When an individual is also struggling with trauma, these deficits are compounded.

However, if one were to draw family diagrams of these individuals, their symptomology would be in keeping with the overall characteristic of the family system. In other words, these individuals are highly unlikely to stand out when compared with other family members over multiple generations, although they may be the most symptomatic member of their nuclear family. This is why it is important for people to understand the relational patterns of their family of origin and their place within a multigenerational context.

The Negative Effect of Avoidance and Numbing

Of all the symptoms of PTSD, avoidance and numbing account for the largest reason for wives seeking divorce, a fact that is also consistent with the larger literature on divorce. According to research conducted by Galovski and Lyons (2004), the wives and children of veterans whose primary symptom of PTSD was avoidance and numbing "came to believe that the veterans did not care for them at all," (p. 483). This finding was corroborated by a meta-analysis of research done on PTSD and intimate relationship problems conducted by Taft, Watkins, Stafford, Street & Monson (2011). They report, "Some preliminary work suggests that avoidance and numbing PTSD symptoms are particularly associated with poor relationship satisfaction," (p. 29).

Moreover, several studies have shown that families of veterans exhibiting avoidance and numbing were less likely to attend family therapy (Galovski and Lyons, 2004, p. 492). Meis, Kehle, Barry, Erbes & Polusny (2010) (in their study of PTSD and treatment utilization among coupled National Guard soldiers) found that those families in which the soldier had lower levels of PTSD symptomology were least likely to seek counseling. While they were not able to draw any firm conclusions, it may be that avoidance and numbing are most prominent at lower levels of PTSD symptomology as these defense mechanisms would mitigate the awareness of distress among the soldiers and their spouses. Thus not only does avoidance and numbing create problems for the relationship, it also contributes to the minimization of the problems themselves by the couple and other family members, making it far less likely that will seek help in a timely manner.

How Couples Accommodate to PTSD

Given our increasing knowledge about the effects of PTSD on couples, little has been written about how to incorporate this understanding into what can be done to address the issues these couples face. One study, however, offers some direction. In research done on couples in which one partner has experienced trauma, Henry, Smith et al (2011) found that couples tended to accommodate to the symptoms of PTSD in five identifiable patterns: the role in relationship, boundary issues, intimacy problems, triggers and coping mechanisms (pp. 325-328). For example, some spouses responded by taking on the role of support, helping to soothe their partner during times of high anxiety. Others took on an instrumental role, seeking specific actions to address issues related to the trauma (pp. 324-325). These roles were most often identified by the partners as direct responses to the challenges of living with PTSD.

These roles, in turn, are maintained by the establishment boundary systems within a framework of rules and patterns of interactions. One example of this is the pursuer-distancer pattern: a common marital problem but one that is uniquely constituted in these couples as the partner with PTSD takes on the tendency to distance in order to protect them from emotional pain and the other seeks to engage their partner. Testing the relationship was also a common characteristic as the partner with PTSD tests to see if their spouse remains committed to the relationship. And here, too, avoidance emerged as a key factor. "Participants discussed avoiding particular issues by pretending that the issues did not exist or impact their lives," they explain (Henry, Smith et al, 2011, p. 326). These boundary patterns contribute to problems with both emotional and sexual intimacy while triggers make it difficult for partners with PTSD to navigate daily relationships.

The Changeable Nature of the Brain

Despite the obstacles to couples struggling with the impact of trauma, the good news is that the human brain is changeable. As Hanson (2013) explains, "The brain is the organ that *learns*, so it is designed to be changed by experiences" (p. 10). Thus, even though one's brain has been affected by trauma, repeated conscious effort over time will change the existing neuropathways, in a process known as experience-dependent neuroplasticity (Hanson, 2013, p. 10). For couples, this means that both partners can work within the relationship to change the emotional valence from reactivity to responsivity. From being driven by the reactivity of the fight, flight, or freeze mechanism to being guided by thoughtful intention and one's deeply held values.

This involves learning to settle one's reactions in order to more accurately evaluate the environment and one's own emotional state and to evaluate the emotional state of others. As van der Kolk (2014) explains, the capacity to allow our pre-frontal cortex (where our thinking takes place) to modulate our reactions is "crucial for preserving our relationships with our fellow human beings," (p. 62).

All coupleships offer the opportunity to grow and change one's brain physiology. However, those couples in which one individual is suffering from PTSD face a unique challenge in that the symptoms of PTSD can best be ameliorated by psychotherapy. In light of this, the partner suffering from the effects of trauma must be engaged in individual psychotherapy with a well-trained mental health professional. This will set the stage for more effective changes within the relationship and allow both partners to focus on shifting patterns so that the relationship works better for both of them.

Making Changes Within the Relationship by Keeping the Focus on Yourself

Addressing the common challenges of couples in general will help to create a roadmap to avoid getting lost in the "weeds" of the details and instead focus on patterns of interaction. Looking at these typical patterns and then changing your part in those patterns allows you to focus on what you can change and helps you avoid focusing on your partner and trying to get him or her to change.

In fact, the primary principle of making positive changes within a relationship is to keep the focus on yourself and avoid becoming focused on your partner. This requires you to be aware of your level of anxiety and to practice responding to situations based on your principles and values. Hard work, but it can be done!

Common Relationship Patterns

There are several patterns that are common to all relationships, but the two that are most identifiable are: pursuer-distancer and overfunctioner-underfunctioner. In the pursuer-distancer dynamic, one partner will react to relational intensity by becoming emotionally distant in an unconscious attempt to prevent the relationship from getting too intense. In response, their partner will begin pushing for more connection in an effort to keep the relationship from getting too cold. Either partner can change their part in this pattern, but usually the pursuer is in the best position to make a change since it is easier to stop doing something (anxiously pursuing) then to start. Whether or not both partners decide to change, each has a part in maintaining this pattern and thus can make changes. The pursuer can learn to recognize when there are increasing levels of conflict in an effort to get their partner to respond. Instead, they can work to lower their anxiety, taking time to settle themselves down, and then respond to their partner with a calm, curiosity about their thinking. The distancer can observe how and when they tend to pull away emotionally, and then decide to initiate a discussion about the issue rather than sweeping things under the rug, hoping the issues will go away.

In the overfunctioner-underfunctioner reciprocity, one partner responds to anxiety by doing more (overfunctioning) and, in response to this, the other partner decreases the amount they do (underfunctioning). Usually the overfunctioner complains that they are doing too much, but is certain that if they don't do it, nobody else will. The underfunctioner, on the other hand, sees the overfunctioner as overly anxious and controlling. They typically complain that the overfunctioner has unrealistic expectations and are never satisfied with any efforts made to assist. Here, too, the key is to lower one's anxious reactivity and respond out of a value or a principle instead. For the overfunctioner, the goal is not to get other people to do more but rather to shift to doing the right amount. This shift would involve a thoughtful discussion with their partner and explore his or her thinking on the topic. Likewise, the underfunctioner can observe their part in this pattern. Perhaps they underfunction in response to their partner's anxiety about doing things the "right" way. If that is the case, then a discussion concerning how much is enough would be a useful one. Underfunctioners often react in an effort to avoid conflict so moving toward one's spouse with thoughtful curiosity will begin to shift this pattern.

Replacing Emotional Reactivity with Thoughtful Intention

It is easy to slip into the above noted patterns because they are not a result of a conscious decision, but reactions to long established relational dynamics in the family of origin. When an event is experienced as similar to one of these older patterns, people react in a way that has been so ingrained that most of the time people are not even aware that this is occurring. Usually people believe that if their partner would change, everything would work out well. If the underfunctioner would just pick up his functioning (usually in the way the overfunctioner wants it to be done), then the overfunctioner would not have to change. Of if the pursuer would just stop making a big deal out of nothing (as the distancer is likely to think), then the distancer would not have to change. Seeing the other person as the problem is easy; recognizing our part in the problem is much more difficult and making changes even more so difficult but not impossible. If we see these opportunities as chances for personal growth, then the way becomes easier.

This starts, however, with a review of one's values and ideals. You cannot make changes if you do not know the basis for making those changes. Changes made in an effort to get someone else to change do not last. Changes based on a value or principle do. For example, if you are an overfunctioner in the area of keeping the house clean, you will need to begin with evaluating your own standards and expectations. How much is enough? What is good enough? This should be followed by a discussion with your partner as to what he or she thinks – not in order to get them to change, but to truly explore their thinking. It is hard to overestimate the value of curiosity when it comes to this process of change. When we are truly curious we are not acting out of an agenda but rather out of a desire to understand the other. It's a challenge because sometimes our motives are not clear, even to ourselves, but even just making the attempt will result in changes to the patterns.

Once you have explored your partner's thinking, then you will have a better idea regarding your own position on the issue. To return to the example of keeping house, let's say your partner thinks he does enough of the housework even though you disagree. You could ask him how much work he thinks he does. And what is he observing about your current pattern? He may say that he tries to help but you don't like how he does it and so he backs off. This will let you know that you may want to evaluate your standards. Or he may say that he think he does enough, and you could then ask him for clarification. What does he do to help with the cleaning? How often? Keep in mind that this is not to win the argument but rather to understand him and to gather more accurate information. Just having this discussion without trying to win will change the dynamics. Keep in mind that changes do not need to be large to have a great impact.

When you make changes like this, you are making changes to the neuropathways in your brain. These are lasting changes because they occur in situations that trigger old reactions but in which you're using new responses. These same strategies are helpful with your family of origin relationships and, in fact, these relationships can be a tremendous resource to you since a change in one relationship will make it easier to change another. You may want to observe, for example, how you overfunction in your family of origin and apply the same principles for change, using thoughtful intention, values-based behavior, and curiosity about the other person.

Lowering Reactivity with Mindfulness Meditation

Becoming aware of your emotional state and your reaction to your environment is the goal of mindfulness meditation. Van der Kolk (2014) has found through his research on trauma that mindfulness meditation helps to repair the "faulty alarm systems" of the brain and restore it to its normal level of functioning (p. 207). "Neuroscience research shows," he explains, "that the only way we can change the way we feel is by becoming aware of our inner experience and learning to befriend what is going on inside ourselves," (p. 208).

Mindfulness meditation, which has its roots in Eastern traditions but is also found in Western Christian contemplative practices, helps people learn to be aware of their emotional experiences without necessarily acting on them. This practice is the best way to lay the foundation for responding to life's challenges with thoughtful intention.

The most common way to establish a mindfulness practice is to set aside a few minutes every day, starting with five minutes, gradually increasing the time to 20 minutes, to sit quietly. You will find that your thoughts seem to be jumbled, jumping from one topic to the next. This is what is called "monkey mind" because your thoughts are like little monkeys jumping from one branch to the next. Just observe your thoughts and let them go, focusing on your breath, and repeating a word such as "peace" or "love." This will allow you to return your attention to your phrase and to your breath as you slowly breathe in and out. In a few minutes, you will find your mind will settle down. You will also find emotions arising. These, too, can be observed and let go. This is not the time to question or investigate; it is a time to be rather than do.

The positive effects of regular meditation practice are cumulative in that they build over time. As a result, you will become less reactive to circumstances that used to set you off before you could think about it. Mindfulness practice can also be combined with physical exercise or yoga and spiritual practices such as contemplative prayer to assist you in creating relationships that are healthier, less emotionally taxing, and more fulfilling.

Conclusion

Most people enter adulthood thinking that they've finished growing up. Nothing could be further from the truth. As we have seen, our lives constantly give us opportunities to learn and grow, to change our relationships and our family systems for the better. The issue of trauma makes this normal process more difficult but not impossible. Rather than allowing the trauma to define them, individuals with PTSD can address their symptoms with a qualified mental health professional while at the same time seek couples therapy to work on relational issues. The result could be a healthier, more fulfilling life than you had ever thought possible and the benefits to you and your family will be passed down through subsequent generations.

References

Galovski, T., & Lyons, J. A. (2004). Psychological sequelae of combat violence: A review of the impact of PTSD on the veteran's family and possible interventions. *Aggression and Violent Behavior*, 477-501.

Hanson, R. (2013). Hardwiring happiness: The new brain science of contentment, calm, and confidence. New York: Harmony Books.

Henry, S. B., Smith, D. B., Archuleta, K. L., Sanders-Hahs, E., Nelson Goff, B. S., Reisbig, K. L., et al. (2011). Trauma and couples: Mechanisms in dyadic functioning. *Journal of Marital and Family Therapy*, 319-332.

Meis, L. A., Kehle, S. M., Barry, R. A., Erbes, C. R., & Polusny, M. A. (2010). Relationship adjustment, PTSD symptoms, and treatment utilization among coupled National Guard soldiers deployed to Iraq. *Journal of Family Psychology*, 560-567.

Schnarch, D. (2009). Passionate marriage: Keeping love and intimacy alive in committed relationships. New York: W.W. Norton & Co.

Taft, C. T., Stafford, J., Watkins, L. E., & Street, A. E. (2011). Posttraumatic stress disorder and intimate relationship problems: A meta-analysis. *Journal of Consulting and Clinical Psychology*, 22-33.

Van der Kolk, B. (2014). The body keeps score: Brain, mind, and body in the healing of trauma. New York: Penguin.

Van der Kolk, B., McFarlane, A. C., & Weisaeth, L. E. (1996). Traumatic Stress: The effects of overwhelming experience on Mind, Body, and Society. New York: Guilford.

Chapter 18 Summary

Vampire Syndrome and
Male Child Sexual Abuse

In Western folklore, a vampire is defined as a corpse that returns from the grave each night to suck the blood from the living. These malignant and malevolent creatures terrorize the inhabitants of the countryside, creating havoc and fragmenting the lives of those with whom they come in contact.

"Vampire syndrome" is a metaphor used to describe the cycle of sexual abuse. Children who are abused are robbed of a part of themselves, and are forever changed into a different person than they would have been. These changes result in a fractured sense of self, manifesting throughout the survivors life, in a multitude of ways such as: internalized anger, loss of control over their behavior, and a lack of self. When a male adult abuses a male child, the survivor tends to adopt a sense of hypermasculinity to compensate for internalized homophobia, and a sense of being "less than a man."

"Vampire syndrome" encompasses the idea of a cause and effect relationship that a male survivor will become an abuser himself. The vampire bites the child, turning him into a vampire, who will then seek out the blood of others, perpetuating a lineage of abuse. This is not only logically faulty, but has been proven false by many studies. If it were true that all survivors – or even most of them – became abusers, then the prevalence would be astronomical. As bad as the rate of abuse is currently, we know the numbers don't support this theory. It also does not account for female victims.

Much of the literature neither argues against, nor supports, the idea that a survivor will become an abuser. There is a possibility and a tendency to become more aggressive and act out in aggressive behavior, but that is a far cry from becoming a child sexual abuser themselves.

Robert has an increased need to protect our son Lawrence. I know one of his greatest fears is our son having to go through what he did as a child. This fear propels a notion in his psyche that he must protect Lawrence, which is normal for a father to want to do. Robert is always well attuned to where Lawrence is and who he is with. Additionally, he is selective of the people he allows around Lawrence. Anyone that exhibits traits that an abuser may potentially carry, like paying too much attention to Lawrence, trying to get too close to him or us, is immediately red-flagged and watched with a careful eye.

Research proves that there are several environmental factors and personality traits that are present in sexual offenders. Childhood abuse is but one of these factors.

Others include childhood exposure to violence and sexual promiscuity.

Studying male survivors has proven to be an arduous and elusive task. It is very difficult to get statistics on the subject due to the lack of reporting of the abuse, and the vehement reluctance to disclose. This is especially true of men who were abused by other males. This group is burdened by warped societal definitions of manhood, and a deep-seated fear of being labeled as a homosexual, or an inferior man. Men who have been abused by women also have a difficult time disclosing, at the risk of being dismissed, laughed off, or ridiculed for not enjoying it.

In folklore, the vampire continues to terrorize the countryside until it is killed – traditionally by stabbing a stake through its heart. For male survivors, their abuse will continue to internally torture them until they put the stake through the trauma by integrating the abuse into their sense of self – thus becoming whole again. Processing and working through the abuse with therapy, self-help groups, or by other means can help a man to achieve this. Childhood abuse fractures the survivor's sense of self, and healing requires and enables the survivor to return to wholeness after the abuse.

Chapter 18

Vampire Syndrome and
Male Child Sexual Abuse

Matthew Love, Psy.D.
Fairfield University

Vampires are thought of individuals who lurk in the shadows and feed on the living. These undead parasitic creatures burst into the English lexicon in 1732 when "vampyre" appeared in English in the London Journalin. The word was used to describe an incident in a rural village of what is now Hungary where a recently deceased villager was dug up a month after his burial and was reportedly undecayed. According to the story, there were reports the villager was harassing his neighbors after his death. The villager was stuck between life and death and thus called "vampyre." The word stuck and ultimately became part of Western culture.

Butz (1993) argues the "vampire syndrome" is a metaphor for Child Sexual Abuse (CSA). He uses the idea that a vampire is an individual who is a corpse and a "different species, sustains immortality through the drinking of blood, the need for blood destroys the victim, and that victims are turned into vampires," (Butz, 1993). Using psychodynamic framework and the vampire as a metaphor for abuse, he illustrates that a victim's body changes following the vampire's attack and it is "only a physical vessel that resembles a human form," (Butz, 1993). It is typical for survivors of CSA to feel a fractured sense of self, dissociation, and overwhelming emotions that manifest months to years after the trauma. Butz (1993) argues the energy exerted to maintain the repressed memory within the unconscious causes the survivor to lose a part of themselves. Since there is no integration of the trauma into the self, the survivor experiences confusion, loss of control over one's behavior, and hyperactivity.

The symbol of blood as fuel for immortality is a metaphor for the transgenerational transmission of abuse that is typically found in family systems where there are young parents who are unable to cope with the high demands of parenthood. Butz (1993) states the metaphor of drinking the blood is the transmission of abuse. The act of abuse or draining the blood of the victim destroys the soul of the survivor as he or she is no longer whole but fractured and searching for meaning. Butz (1993) does not argue that if a child is sexually abused, he or she will become an abuser. He does state that there is a "gestation period" where the survivor may become an aggressor if he or she is not returned to whole. Returning to a sense of wholeness relates how the survivor heals after the abuse occurs. The course of healing takes many different paths with various endings.

The question then is how does the vampire myth relate to CSA? As previously described, the idea of vampires is of individuals who lurk in the shadows and feed on the living for their own survival. In essence, the vampire is seen as a creature who indulges in hedonistic behavior with little regard to the other. CSA is ultimately a power-dominant relationship between the perpetrator and survivor where the survivor is manipulated emotionally, physically, and sexually to satisfy a non-sexual desire of power and dominance for the perpetrator. Within a CSA relationship the perpetrator objectifies, similar to the way the vampire objectifies the living force in his own survival, the child.

In addition to the vampire's purpose is power and dominance, which is similar to the dynamics found within the CSA relationship. Survivors of sexual abuse often develop the cognitive construct that since they were abused they will then become a perpetrator. Within clinical literature, the idea of the cause and effect relationship between the survivor's becoming a perpetrator is known as the "vampire syndrome." According to O'Brien (1991), prior sexual victimization is a factor for sexual offending. He found that 42% of sexual offenders had been previously sexually victimized by a sibling, which was the highest rate within his study. This supported the findings of Smith and Israel (1987) who found that 52% of sexual offenders had prior sexual victimization.

While there is some evidence that a percentage of perpetrators were exposed to a prior sexual trauma, it is not a strong "cause and effect" link. In an effort to better explain the separation between those who offend and those who do not, Finkelhor (1984) developed *The Four Factor Model* of sexual abuse. The four consistent factors found in perpetrators: (a) the perpetrator is attracted to weak, vulnerable or non-threatening individuals; (b) experiencing sexual arousal to children or young people regardless of social norms; (c) having the ability to overcome the survivor's resistance; and (d) being disinhibited or lacking impulse control (Finkelhor, 1984, Love, 2014). Without these conditions present in an individual's psyche, it is highly unlikely the CSA survivor will engage in offending behavior.

For some time, the idea that prior sexual victimization was the cause for future sexual perpetration was constituent within clinical literature. However, this idea is overly simplistic and also neglects a major question. If prior sexual victimization is necessary for future perpetration, then there must be a single origin for all sexual perpetration/victimization. Logically, we know that one single entity did not create child sexual abuse. There are multiple environmental factors that facilitate the growth of a perpetrator. According to St-Yves and Pellertin's (2002) research with sexual offenders in Canada, prior sexual victimization was not the only cause for sexual offending. There are numerous environmental factors that increased the likelihood of someone becoming a sexual offender. Notably childhood exposure to violence, sexual promiscuity, or substance abuse were found in the etiology of sexual offenders (St-Yves & Pellertin, 2002).

These are important factors when examining the likelihood of sexual offending because they are essential for the development of empathy and emotional reciprocation. The child who is exposed to domestic violence, physical abuse, emotional abuse, sexual abuse, or substance use is less likely to experience a secure attachment with a primary caregiver and less likely to experience appropriate mirroring of emotions from that caregiver. Additionally, what we see in these family dynamics are low parental supervision, which leads to a poor understanding of interpersonal boundaries because children are not provided with an adequate understanding of pro-social behavior. Thus, sexual offending can occur within a family dynamic where sexual abuse was absent.

St-Yves and Pellerin (2002) point out that 50% of individuals who committed a sex crime were not sexual abused as children. The vampire syndrome does not explain the reason that many who were sexual abused as children do not abuse others. St-Yves and Pellerin (2002) argue the tendency by those who perpetrate CSA to rationalize their behavior by amplifying or creating prior trauma to reduce the internalized shame and guilt for their actions.

Thus far we have spent some time examining the development of the "vampire syndrome" and exploring the validity of the assumption that perpetrators of CSA were previously abused. It is an overly simplistic view to a rather complex relationship between interpersonal, environmental, and social factors that influence how a survivor integrates the trauma experience into one's sense of self. Regardless of the survivor's gender, CSA is damaging to one's psyche because of relationship with the perpetrator. CSA is not an abrupt single incident trauma but rather a series of subtle interpersonal boundary violations enacted by the perpetrator to desensitizing the child to the ultimate act of sexual contact. This is known as "grooming," and the perpetrator not only grooms the child but the environment and caregivers by creating a trustworthy façade (Salter, 1995; McAlinden, 2006; van Dam, 2011). As a result, the fractured sense of self for the CSA survivor is amplified because at the heart of the sexual trauma is a betrayal of trust due to coercion, manipulation, and sexual exploitation by the perpetrator (Brackenridge, 2001; Finkelhor & Browne, 1988; Spiegel, 2003; van Dam, 2001; Wekerle & Wolfe, 2003). As previously mentioned, this leads to a sense of confusion and search for meaning on the part of the survivor to return to whole.

Male survivors of CSA are historically underrepresented in clinical literature due to lack of reporting. Less than 10% of CSA cases are disclosed to authorities, which creates a dearth of research (Goodyear-Brown, Fath, Myers, 2012). Male survivors face a daunting task for disclosure when the perpetrator is also male due to the survivor experiencing internalized homophobia and societal beliefs of masculinity (Hartill, 2005; Walker, Archer, & Davies, 2005; Valente, 2005; Alaggia & Millington, 2008; Alaggia, 2005; Nalavany & Abell, 2004; Lisak, 1994; Sageman, 2003; Love, 2014).

Boys learn from a young age that to be a man means to be powerful and dominant. Within Western culture, masculinity is the avoidance of overt expressions of femininity. The suppression of feminine characteristics peaks between the ages of 5 and 7 years old (Kohlberg, 1966; Martin, Ruble, & Szkrybalo, 2002). This coincides with the typical age of the onset of CSA and likely creates an internal conflict for the male survivor because he has an experience (i.e. submitting to the will of another) goes against societal beliefs of what it means to be masculine (Love, 2014). At such a young age, the child does not understand the nuances of the relationship. Specifically, he does not understand that he was manipulated by another rather than being a willingly participant.

The male survivor is left feeling empty, confused, and desperate to define the experience within his masculine worldview. As a result, the male survivor often believes the perpetrator knew he was gay. This belief is often wrongly confirmed by the male survivor because he experienced arousal and at times ejaculated. The thought the male survivor has that "if I experienced an erection and/or ejaculated than I must have enjoyed the sexual contact." As a young child, the male survivor is unable to separate what is a physiological response to that of pleasure. The avoidance of the trauma and belief he must be gay because the survivor was abused by a male perpetrator magnifies his loss of identity. In an effort to reclaim a sense of self, the male survivor typically adopts an ultra-conservative view of masculinity known as hyper-masculinity that epitomizes the ideal aspects of the Western man (i.e. power and dominance).

As the male survivor retreats further into his hyper-masculine worldview, he experiences increasingly internal discomfort due to an internalized homonegativity. The child begins to experience an internalized negative relationship towards himself due to the possibility of being gay. Children experience this concept because their foundation of who they are, is destroyed. The child is attempting to make sense of why he was chosen by the perpetrator, thus attempting to regain power over an imbalanced relationship. The more he attempts to regain power, the more his confusion around his sexual orientation grows. He believes the perpetrator must have known he was gay and that would have been the only reason he would have engaged the child in a sexual relationship.

Following the unwanted sexual contact by a man, the child is left shattered and looking for a sense of direction. His childhood is robbed and the male child experiences difficulty defining who he is after the unwanted sexual experience. The experience falls into social taboo and he feels alone to navigate this new arena in which he was unprepared. In an effort to regain control, power, and dominance over his life, the male child seeks to define who he is within the world. Without proper therapeutic intervention, he may develop the concept that he must have wanted to interaction to occur otherwise he would have done something to stop it. The male child develops false beliefs as to who he will become in an effort make sense of who he is after the abuse occurred. Without a proper integration of the abuse into his sense of self, it will continue to live on and terrorize (i.e. vampire) the male child.

References

Alaggia, R. (2005). Disclosing the trauma of child sexual abuse: A gender analysis. *Journal of Loss and Trauma, 10,* 453-470. doi: 10.1080/15320500193895

Alaggia, R., & Millington, G. (2008). Male child sexual abuse: A phenomenology of betrayal. *Clinical Social Work Journal, 36*(3), 265-275. doi:10.1007/s10615- 007-0144-y

Brackenridge, C. (2001). *Spoilsports: Understanding and preventing sexual exploitation in sport.* London; New York; United Kingdom: Routledge.

Bütz, M. R. (1993), THE VAMPIRE AS A METAPHOR FOR WORKING WITH CHILDHOOD ABUSE. American Journal of Orthopsychiatry, 63: 426-431. doi:10.1037/h0079449

Finkelhor, D. (1984). *Child sexual abuse: New theory and research.* New York: Free Press.

Finkelhor, D., & Browne, A. (1988). Assessing the long-term impact of child abuse: A review and conceptualization. In L. Walker (Ed.), *Handbook on sexual Abuse of children* (pp. 55-71). New York: Springer.

Goodyear-Brown, P., Fath, A., & Myers, L. (2012). *Child sexual abuse: The scope of the* problem. In Goodyear-Brown, P. (Eds.), *Handbook of child sexual abuse: Identification, assessment, and treatment* (3-10). Hoboken, NJ: John Wiley & Sons.

Hartill, M. (2005). Sport and the sexually abused male child. *Sport, Education and Society, 10*(3), 287-304, doi: 10.1080/13573320500254869

Kohlberg, L. A. (1996). A cognitive-development analysis of children's sex role concepts and attitudes. In E. E. Maccoby (Eds.), *Toward a feminist development of sex differences* (p. 82-173). Stanford, CA: Stanford University Press.

O'Brien, M. J. (1991). Taking sibling incest seriously. In M. Q. Patton (Ed.), *Family sexual abuse: Frontline research and evaluation.* (pp. 75-92). Newbury Park, CA.: Sage Publications.

Lisak, D. (1994). The psychological impact of sexual abuse: Content analysis of interviews with male survivors. *Journal of Traumatic Stress, 7*(4), 525-548. doi: 10.1002/jts.2490070403

Love, M. (2014). *Sexual abuse of male children in sports: Factors impacting disclosure* (Doctoral dissertation).

McAlinden, A.-M. (2006). 'Setting 'Em Up': Personal, Familial and Institutional Grooming in the Sexual Abuse of Children. Social & Legal Studies, 15, 339-62.

Martin, C. L., Ruble, D. N., & Szkrybalo. J. (2002). Cognitive theories of early gender development. *Psychological Bulletin, 128*(6), 903-933. doi: 10.1037//0033-2909.128.6.903

Nalavany, B. A., & Abell, N. (2004). An initial validation of a measure of personal And social perceptions of the sexual abuse of males. *Research on Social Work in Practice, 14*(5), 368-378. doi: 10.1177/1049731504265836

Sageman, S. (2003). The rape of boys and the impact of sexually predatory environments: Review and case reports. *Journal of the American Academy of Psychoanalysis, 31*(3), 563-580.

  doi: 10.1521/jaap.31.3.563.22137

St-Yves, M. & Pellerin, B. (2002). Sexual victimization and sexual delinquency: Vampire or Pinocchio syndrome? Correctional Service Canada Forum, 14, 51-52.

Salter, A.C. (1992). *Transforming Trauma: A Guide to Understanding and Treating Adult Survivors of Child Sexual Abuse.* Los Angeles: SAGE Publications, Inc; 1 edition

Valente, S. M. (2005). Sexual abuse of boys. *Journal of Child and Adolescent Psychiatric Nursing, 18*(1), 10-16. doi: 10.1111/j.1744-6171.2005.00005.x

van Dam, C. (2001). *Identifying child molesters: Preventing child sexual abuse by recognizing the patterns of the offenders.* New York: Haworth Maltreatment and Trauma Press.

Walker, J., Archer, J., & Davies, M. (2005). Effects of rape on men: A descriptive analysis. *Archives of Sexual Behavior, 34*(1), 69-80. doi: 10.1007/s10508-1001-0

Wekerle, C. & Wolfe, D. A. (2003). Child maltreatment. In E. J. Mash, & R.A. Barkley (Eds.), *Child psychopathology* (2nd ed., pp. 632-683). New York: Guilford Press.

Chapter 19 Summary

Perspectives of The Battered Man: Psychology, Neurobiology, Male Conditioning, and Recommendations

Domestic abuse/violence is a problem with many different aspects. One of the least talked about parts of domestic violence is the fact that men can be targets. Usually the discussion centers on men as the perpetrators, due to the size and power imbalance in a stereotypical male/female heterosexual relationship.

What is not often discussed is the emotional power imbalance where men feel disempowered as a full participant in the relationship. This is what my husband experienced with his first marriage. The power and control that his wife exerted over him with her constant supervision and suspicion that he was cheating on her was an emotional dominance that robbed him of his sense of self.

This chapter delves deeply into the world of domestic violence, how it affects men and women, what we can do to help men recover from the negative effects and prevent them from repeating the negative relationship behaviors that led to the choices they made.

As an overview of the universe of domestic violence from many different sides, this chapter covers the social science as well as the neuroscience behind the long-term damage suffered by a survivor of domestic violence. Many times, a survivor of domestic violence or abuse will exhibit symptoms of post-traumatic stress disorder such as anxiety, hypervigilance, depression, and suicidal ideations. For male survivors this can be especially devastating to their sense of self, for society tells them that as a man they should be strong, silent, and able to overcome their problems by themselves. The truth is that for males who are survivors, they have to overcome not just the immediate effects of the abuse or violence, but also rebuild their ego and self-esteem as men, just as women do, though in a system that is not supportive of them and their struggles.

Chapter 19

Perspectives of The Battered Man: Psychology, Neurobiology, Male Conditioning, and Recommendations

Michael Levittan Ph.D.
Private Practice

In 21st century Western societies, there are well-established and familiar "coming-out-of-the-closet" phenomena related to the rights of women, minorities, gays, and children. For the vast majority of human history, there has been prejudice, abuse, and various forms of atrocity perpetuated behind closed doors and swept under the rug. Beginning with animal abuse and then child abuse, there have been activists, movements, media stories, fictionalized accounts, and finally legislation and law enforcement that serve to enlighten society, develop laws, and initiate treatment programs designed to address these issues.

In the field of domestic violence, it is both assumed and documented that, for the most part, men are perpetrators and women represent the abused. Data from prestigious organizations such as the Department of Justice, the American Bar Association, the World Health Organization, the Centers for Disease Control, and the National Coalition Against Domestic Violence are all reflective of the strong tendency to ascribe perpetration to men. Most batterers' treatment programs in the U.S. use various modifications of a psycho-educational, feminist curriculum, and many domestic violence organizations have a strong bias against empathizing with the male perspective.

A personal bias also needs to be stated here. When referencing one's own group, whether it be designated by profession, race, sexual orientation, or gender, arguments tend to fall into one of two polar opposite positions: either you promote your group and extol its virtues, or the misdeeds and bad behaviors of certain members of your group makes you feel shame for being associated with them. As a man, I acutely feel ashamed for the stereotypical (but very real) bad behaviors of some men, such as the braggarts, loudmouths, fighters, intimidators, abusers, and perpetrators of violence. I find those men who use their size and strength to take advantage of physically weaker individuals, as well as men on a perennial quest to prove and assert their manhood, to be particularly difficult to stomach. At times, it even feels as if I bear some degree of responsibility for the behavior of all men. My feelings may not all seem logical, but they have been present as far back as I can remember.

Therefore, it is a challenge to be open-minded enough to write this chapter from the perspective of men who are themselves victims of domestic violence. Our brain abhors uncertainty, so human beings tend to quickly and automatically categorize stimuli. When we label something and put it in a box, we are – at least temporarily – removing the uncertainty. To re-label categories or create new ones takes the mental and emotional work of reevaluating long established, monolithic concepts. This reevaluation is a prerequisite to an exploration of what men experience when they are abused by their partners.

Definitions

Though violence or the threat of violence is often a key component of domestic violence, it ultimately involves more than a single incident. Domestic violence represents a pattern in an intimate relationship where one person actively seeks to establish and maintain power and control over their partner. Dr. Mary Ann Dutton defines it as: "A pattern of interaction in which one intimate partner is forced to change his or her behavior in response to threats or abuse from their partner," (1994). According to California state law, spousal battery involves: "Intentionally or recklessly causing or attempting to cause bodily injury to a family or household member, or date, or placing a family or household member, or date, in reasonable apprehension of imminent serious bodily injury to him/herself or another," (CA. Penal Code 273.5 or 243[e]).

Biases in Domestic Violence Data

Most recent studies report that males are predominantly the perpetrators of domestic violence. When we consider that the vast majority of samples of data are collected from court-mandated batterers' treatment programs, police reports, women's shelters, and emergency rooms, the conclusions drawn would obviously have an asymmetric bias with regard to perpetration. Men also seem to experience more shame than women about reporting abuse, so this serves as an additional factor in the dearth of reporting and research on male victims (Mulroney and Chan, 2008). In a great majority of cases, shelters provide services to women with male partners and batterers' treatment programs are targeted at men who abuse women. With regard to police arrests made in domestic violence situations, the assumption remains that the man has committed violence against the woman (Cook, 2009). Men are more apt to run and flee the scene, which leaves only the woman to tell her side of the story. It is likely also true that the male-dominated, masculine ethos existing in police departments renders it more difficult for officers arriving on the scene to view a man as the victim in a violent domestic altercation.

The issue of underreporting domestic violence is quite prevalent for both genders. Men and women often seek to protect their partners from incarceration and it is quite significant that there exists ongoing fear of the consequences of revealing the abuse to anyone. The "behind closed doors" privacy issue for family matters has prevailed for most of recorded history and is a powerful factor in underreporting. Though shame is usually experienced for both men and women when making violence known outside the bounds of the relationship, men tend to feel the shame more acutely than women. The issue of shame as it relates to male conditioning is discussed later in this chapter.

Actual data from various studies and surveys provides somewhat contradictory conclusions regarding domestic violence victims and perpetrators by gender. According to recent data from the Centers for Disease Control and Prevention (2013), domestic violence victims are surprisingly near equal in terms of gender. At least 40% of victims in the United States are male (CDC, 2013) and approximately one in four men experience intimate partner violence each year.

Differences are more sharply drawn when we consider the severity of physical abuse, as approximately 22% of women have been a victim of severe physical abuse in an intimate relationship, while approximately 14% of men have experienced the same (CDC, 2014). Noted researcher Murray Straus reports that in intimate and dating relationships, women are about half as likely as men are to perpetrate severe abuse (2011).

Incidents of homicide in intimate relationships seem to hold steady year after year, with approximately 1,250 murder victims being female and 450 being male. When women are murdered, 33% of the time it is at the hands of a partner. For men who are murdered, 4% are victimized by their partner. Men commit about six times as many homicides as women do, but they also account for four times as many victims of homicide. It must be acknowledged that when it comes to actual physical and gun-related violence, males are most often the perpetrator.

Worldwide, the largest category for homicide consists of male-on-male violence.

Putting aside gender comparisons, domestic violence appears to be an intractable problem in the United States. Taking the continual, vast underreporting of abuse into account, the issue for both genders has reached epidemic proportions in our so-called civilized society. It is factual reality that adult males have perpetrated and continue to perpetrate the majority of overall violence. However, this reality must not detract from the often neglected, but quite relevant reality that men also represent the majority of victims of violence and that this victimhood for violence often begins when these same men were little boys.

Gender Differences with Anger and Aggression

When aggression and violence are viewed purely from an instinctual, evolutionary perspective, it clearly follows that males propagate their genes only by gaining access to sexually-fertile females. Therefore, it holds that throughout the generations young females in the prime of their reproductive life are the most frequent victims of male aggression and violence. Disparity in size and strength exacerbate the issue of male violence toward females. Correlations between sexual dimorphism and male aggression can be observed in most species. Generally, humans exhibit less dimorphism (males weigh approximately 12% more than females) than chimpanzees (males weigh twice as much as females) and elephant seals (males weigh four times as much as females).

In addition to advantages in size and weight, human males often have more experience in athletics and physical combat.

Therefore, most men have the ability - even without the use of aggression or violence - to present their physicality in an imposing, intimidating manner. People react to each other on levels of cognition, emotion, and relationship history. Humans also share many traits with other mammalian species, and like animals we react on the primitive level of instinct and survival. When two adults - behind closed doors - are in a conflict and in close proximity, an obvious disparity on physical presence is experienced by both parties. As part of our survival instinct, the "weaker" individual is especially conscious of the disparity. Advantage: males.

Many studies have been done for the purpose of comparing rates of violence and aggression between women and men. The results of studies done on gender aggression are mixed and in some cases quite contradictory. Arnold Buss developed an early questionnaire on aggression and conducted one of the first studies on human aggression (The Psychology of Aggression, 1966). The results revealed that there were few differences in frequency and displays of aggression between women and men. One of the few disparities the study confirmed was that women were more likely than men to cry or deny something to another when they were angry. Both women and men engage in verbal and psychological abuse. Men typically demean other men with degrading remarks about sexual potency, often employing a label of a feminine pejorative. Women tend to degrade other women by smearing them as being sexually promiscuous. Studies also reveal that women are more apt to feel empathy than men, which is likely a prime factor in the fact that women are more restrained when they do use aggression (Frodi, MacCaulay, and Thome, 1977). Both men and women display aggression in intimate relationships with comparable frequency, though men act with aggression more often in public settings (Fitz, 1979; Tavris, 1982).

To further break down the variables of aggression, Bettencourt and Miller (1996) conducted a meta-analysis of the function that provocation plays in acting-out behavior. They found that men are more likely to interpret provocations more intensely than women and also react more strongly to perceived danger from retaliation. Reactions to real or perceived provocations are no doubt a main factor in the vast disparity in same-sex aggression. Over the years, data on differences in aggression by gender show the greatest disparity in same-sex violence. No matter the historical era, cultural context, or ages involved, male on male violence as well as homicide, is a rampant problem that remains largely unaddressed.

For all children, observing and experiencing family violence has lasting effects and sets a model for adult relationships. In addition to his notable work on trauma, van der Kolk (1989) studied the correlation between early identifications and aggression. He found definite tendencies for abused boys to identify with the aggressive caretaker and become aggressors themselves, while girls tend to attach to aggressive, abusive men and become victims.

It is interesting to note that women tend to score higher on perpetration of domestic violence when data is gathered by self-report. In his study, "Examining Gender Differences in Nature and Context of Intimate Partner Violence" (2012), Hyunkag Cho found that women reported that they perpetrated violence in higher rates than men reported. Perhaps, this is reflective of the greater shame that men experience. With regard to severity of violence, women and men reported approximately equal rates of perpetration.

More recently, researchers emphasize the importance of distinguishing among different types of violence in intimate relationships. Michael Johnson, in his journal article "Conflict and Control: Gender Symmetry and Asymmetry in Domestic Violence" (2006), distinguishes between different types of couples' violence. Defending oneself or reacting to an attack is called situational or responsive violence, and Johnson found relative symmetry with regard to women and men. In terms of "intimate terrorism," the coercive control of a partner, he found this to be the main province of men. While Johnson acknowledges that women do initiate violence, he maintains that for the most part, women engage in "violent resistance" against their partner's aggression. The New York State Office for the Prevention of Domestic Violence (http://opdv.ny.gov/faqs/index.html#maleandfemaleper ps) uses the term "responsive violence" on the part of women in drawing a distinction from the ongoing, controlling nature of male violence.

Emotional Processing and Neurobiology Differences
Gender conditioning begins early in life, sometimes prior to birth. Prospective parents may paint the coming newborn girl's room pink and boy's room blue, with baby clothes picked out in keeping with this distinction. Studies show that parents speak more about sadness with their daughters, and more about anger with their sons (Pollack, 1998). When parents of school-age children dispense their words of wisdom on dealing with situations of conflict, the advice given tends to be polar opposite in nature: for girls, they are instructed to reestablish harmony, to make peace; for boys, the advice is to seek retaliation, to fight back, with an accompanying tone of admonishment. Parenting is a key factor in determining levels of aggression, as recent studies show it is not so much a boy's testosterone level that makes him aggressive, but more about the caretakers who shape his behaviors (Pollack, 1998).

Brain research on gender difference reveal specific disparities between males and females involving thought, emotion, and behavior. Allowing for generalizations, overall, women tend to be better able to process emotions (Kret, M. and DeGelder, B., 2012). This processing enables females to be faster and more accurate at identification and expression of feelings, as well as having less difficulty controlling emotions. The female advantage in emotional processing is often characterized as women possessing higher levels of an "empathizing brain," with the males having higher levels of a "systematizing brain" (Nettle, 2007; Baron-Cohen, 2009). Women prove to be more adept at both encoding facial differences and determining vocal intonations. In totality, women seem to be better able to observe and identify another person's emotions and needs, and then allow these feelings and needs to resonate within (be "touched"). Emotionally understanding another person typically allows for more appropriate responses, and thus greater social connection. The systematizing brain, where males possess higher levels, may confer advantages in exploring, analyzing, and even constructing a system. Men seem better able to make use of thought and intuition to figure out a system, extract the underlying rules that govern the dynamics of that system, and thus predict behaviors and invent a new system.

The neurobiology underlying these sex differences have a basis in brain scans showing that men generally have greater intra-hemispheric connectivity, allowing for more focused attention on tasks. Women tend to have greater inter-hemispheric connectivity, which allows for more flexibility in switching from the logical left brain to the feeling-oriented right brain (Ingalhalikar, M, et. al., 2014). The corpus callosum, connecting the hemispheres, shows increased thickness (connectivity) for females as early as the fetal stage of development. To further the argument that empathy is a more female-oriented faculty, neuroscience research reveals that women listen to others using both left and right hemispheres, while men only employ the right hemisphere when listening (Lurito, 2001).

Females seem to have several innate advantages in the ability to control aggression. In addition to a greater capacity for empathy, which is a prime inhibitor of aggression, girls develop language skills more quickly than boys. Therefore, they are more likely to communicate with words rather than actions, and have greater facility verbalizing their wants and needs. Girls also reach puberty two years earlier than boys. Consequently, it is well established that the prefrontal cortex develops earlier in girls compared to boys. The prefrontal cortex, governing the executive functions of the brain, serves to thoughtfully consider the consequences of our actions and inhibit impulses for aggression. Though there may well be evolutionary advantages to an innate male drive to action and aggression, it certainly makes for more difficulties during both childhood and adulthood to manage the inevitable aggressive impulses that arise for all people.

Male Conditioning and its Enforcers

Conditioning that is grounded in the relational and social aspects of one's society is a normal part of child development for girls and boys. The internalization of modeled behavior, thought patterns and attitudes toward culture and gender occurs both within the family unit and in the greater society. As mentioned previously, gender roles are separate and rigidly defined early in life. For males, that separate role may well be defined more rigidly, with harsher penalties for disobedience, than for females (Begley, 2000).

Throughout generations and cultures, there appears to be conspicuous differences in child-rearing of boys versus girls. Traditionally, girls are more often raised to be responsible for younger siblings and look after others. Also, mothers tend to engage in more detailed reminiscing about emotional events with daughters, in comparison to sons, which might facilitate female capacities for perceiving and being attuned to the inner states of others. In childhood, the more ruminative style of girls brings the tendency to engage in inward forms of aggression (sadness, cutting), while boys typically display more outwardly directed means of aggression. Boys have a definite tendency to internalize the behavior of their father, where conflict is likely to be resolved through action.

Additionally, males in Western society typically inculcate traits of competition, aggression, independence, and dominance. Anderson (2013), in his discussion of male socialization, mentioned the importance of being perceived as powerful, resolute, and self-reliant. Along with strong pressures to attain these masculine traits, there exists an implicit attempt to exclude qualities of discussion, emotion, vulnerability, and reminiscing.

Most young males live in environments where misogynistic attitudes and exemplars of ultra-masculinity are idealized. Boys who exhibit qualities of femininity, passivity, and vulnerability are scorned. Tools employed by males, young and old, to enforce masculine values include both sexist language and brute force which are designed to punish "soft" boys. The most demeaning words a non-masculine boy is labeled with are pejoratives that are feminine in nature.

Most every adult male has suffered some form of humiliation or brutality in childhood with regard to "failures" of masculinity.

Traumas to the Male Psyche

The parameters established for boys (developing males) are learned and internalized as both crucial and urgent tasks of childhood. From very early in life, male identities are "coded by masculine scripts" (Pearson, 1997). The inevitable failures to attain these initiations into manhood often rise to the threshold of trauma, and can be termed, "Traumas to the Male Psyche." For action-oriented males, each trauma tends to bring about a behavioral response or "antidote" to the trauma. What is most significant is that each attempt by the male to overcome the trauma and attain the sought-after antidote brings another round of shame and disgrace and furthers the drive to prove and assert his manhood. Following are three interrelated traumas and their antidotes:

1) Emasculation: Throughout history and across cultures and religions, there have been formalized rituals meant to initiate boys into the "circle of men." Equally potent as a force on boyhood, are the implicit standards of masculinity established by fathers, peers, and the greater society. Every boy - to varying degrees – goes through their own personal, internal struggle to achieve these standards. When not

meeting masculine standards, young males are not just denied eagerly-sought approval from their father, but also must endure his verbal and facial expressions of opprobrium.

Each real or perceived "failure" is chastised through criticism, shaming, and at times, verbal and physical violence. External degradations of boys are matched by their internal feelings of disgrace.

The antidote to emasculation is "ultra-masculinity," which can be defined as the idealized, lofty status of the man perceived to possess extreme traits of masculinity (physical strength, vast wealth, sexual prowess, powerful position, macho attitude, daring feats of performance, fast cars, etc.). Consequences of striving for ultra-masculine status include behavioral adaptations and inevitable disappointments for not reaching those standards.

2) Closeness with Femininity: Early in life, boys are demeaned and mocked for displaying female mannerisms, playing with girls, or being a "Momma's boy." In reaction, boys learn to explicitly and implicitly reject closeness with females. This rejection manifests in narrowed behavioral, cognitive, and emotional constraints for boys that are diametrically opposed to feminine traits. As a further antidote to contact with the feminine, males begin at an early age to subjugate girls and women. Boys employ verbal put-downs or pull a ponytail, while men may exert control over women through intimidation or physical violence.

3) Contact with Emotionality: Both implicitly and explicitly, newborn males are instructed not to express their

feelings. By expressing feelings or showing sensitivity to feelings, boys are violating the standards of displaying a strict masculine bearing. Boys receive myriad messages on many levels throughout childhood, such as "be a man of action" and "tough it out." Other males, be it paternal figures or peers, often ridicule boys who express "softer" emotions (other than anger to express vulnerability). Pollack (1998) emphasizes that anger is the only really acceptable emotion for boys to express, and the anger becomes their "emotional funnel." The antidote to the trauma of emotionality is to restrict one's range of feelings, to include aggression and exclude vulnerability.

Feminist Perspectives on Domestic Violence

Feminists, as well as many men, maintain that domestic violence is "deeply gendered" (Marin and Russo, 1999). This means that violence in relationships is not merely a conflict tactic used to gain the upper hand in the immediate conflict or argument that the couple is engaging in, but that violence is a means of coercion with the intent being to gain control over one's partner and attain the top position in the power hierarchy. When we factor in the physical advantages that men typically possess and display, a legitimate case can be made that women use violence as a means of self-defense. Women may fight back in order to protect themselves from imminent violence by their spouse, or they may retaliate for past abuse inflicted on them, whether physical or psychological. Any human being who has been a long-term victim of aggressive, controlling behavior has the capacity to react with violence at some point. Therefore, the feminist perspective includes the concept that women arrested for domestic violence more typically fit the profile of female victim than male batterer. The perspective does acknowledge that some women do have anger problems, which can be accompanied by violent outbursts.

Male Perspectives on Domestic Violence

When it comes to the very real and "inflammatory" topic of domestic violence, men are typically hyperaware of society's immediate attribution of perpetration to the male. Consequently, men involved in domestic violence incidents feel that their version of events – as well as their feelings - will be ignored by the public, particularly the legal justice system. Men often believe that the legal system is biased against them and they will not be given a "fair shake." It seems that every crisis endured and/or caused by human beings brings with it controversial myths involving the designation of blame and responsibility. In the last two decades, there exists the myth – spread far and wide by the public and even the police – that the failure to effectively prosecute O.J. has caused a "crackdown" on men by legislatures and law enforcement.

Both women and men often automatically view the male as the perpetrator, and in fact men do perpetrate the majority of domestic violence crimes. Yet, to fully understand the psyche of the 21st century man, it is important to recognize that anger and aggression may be covering and shielding deeper feelings of guilt, shame, insecurity, failure, and the sense that when it comes to domestic violence, he is already "behind the eight ball."

What must also be considered is that many men have witnessed acts of aggression, abuse, or physical violence perpetrated by their fathers against their mothers. For boys who endure the experience of violence committed by their idealized paternal object, the impact and the images internalized at the time, both consciously and unconsciously, are still existent in their present-day psyches. Men may well have persistent feelings of guilt for their father's transgressions or guilt for any of their own acts of aggression. Some men are also haunted by guilt over the omnipresent acts of aggression perpetrated by men in general, including violence, bullying, torture, and rape. The seemingly incessant violence committed by males can bring the experience of shame for just being a man.

Society's Attitudes toward Male Victims

Society recognizes and memorializes men's violence against women much more than women's violence toward men (Lupri, E.; Grandin, E., 2014). In his landmark book *Abused Men* (2009), Philip Cook states that the public appears to deplore wife abuse, while treating husband abuse as a humorous topic. Ghanim (2012), in his essay on gender violence, states that: "Female violence is neglected in gender literature...the widespread dominance of male violence in society leaves little room for attending to female violence" (p. 61). Stereotypes prevail that men are aggressive and violent in nature. Pollack (1998) postulated that early in boyhood, males are branded as dangerous and must be watched and kept under strict control.

It requires openness of mind and reevaluation of belief to realistically consider the fact that adult males can be abused in their relationships. Well-established beliefs do not easily change, so society pays scant attention to research on male victims. Studies of this nature are severely lacking, in part because many government agencies refuse to recognize the problem and provide funds for research (Cook, 2009; Wright, 2016). Additionally, there is a lack of resources for male victims, including hotline responses, men's shelters, and treatment programs. It was not until 2016 that the first men's shelter in the United States opened in Alabama. If men victimized by domestic violence do decide to seek support and housing, they must typically reach out to homeless shelters. There exist many documented accounts that describe male help-seekers who have been ignored, doubted, ridiculed, given false information, referred to batterers' treatment programs, and even arrested (Cook, 2009). These failures of service for battered men impact their physical and mental health and exacerbate feelings of isolation and helplessness that are common to any victim of domestic violence.

Impact of Partner Violence on Male Victims

In addition to physical injuries suffered and possibly visible bandages and bruises for family, friends, and work associates to see, the man victimized by domestic violence often endures feelings of shame, guilt, increased anxiety, diminished self-esteem, and self-loathing. Tangible consequences of intimate partner violence may include loss of job, home, relationship, and contact with children. Secondary effects include the use or abuse of alcohol and drugs to escape from these feelings and losses.

As with women victims, there is the loss of safety and trust in one's partner. These essential losses - in post-traumatic fashion – begin to take effect beyond the confines of the family and extend to the lack of safety and trust in the world at-large. Symptoms of PTSD are often present, including severe anxiety, flashbacks, isolation, hypervigilance with regard to one's environment (manifesting in the "walking on eggshells" phenomenon), and traumatic reenactments. It no longer feels safe to express oneself, so the consequent repression of affect brings about depression, along with unexpressed and unresolved anger. As so often occurs with PTSD, the thoughts and feelings engendered by the original incident soon prevail over all aspects of a person's life.

Depression is an obvious mental state for any victim of a crime. When recounting events to others, there are usually statements of blame of others, but internally the victim inevitably blames him or herself. Perhaps, to retain a sense of "control" over the situation, victims tend to attribute a variety of self-deprecatory motives to themselves. As victims wonder how they ever landed in this seemingly inescapable situation, they become filled with self-blame, which may be accompanied by self-loathing, impulses to self-harm, as well as suicidal ideation.

States of depression also can persist for men who feel that they failed in their role as a husband, father, and real man. The perceived loss of masculine status and diminishment in standing or power can result in problems of sexual dysfunction and impotence. The enduring nature of many of these traumatic symptoms can remain in the psyche for a lifetime.

Obstacles to Reporting Abuse

For both genders, there exist both real and psychological challenges for victims of abuse to speak up about the situation, let alone make a report to the authorities. We live in a world where "keeping up appearances" is a major priority for many people. Therefore, the already felt shame and anticipated future shame drives victims to bear the situation and make continual attempts to rationalize or even deny the abuse. Reporting abuse to authorities may feel tantamount to ending the relationship. Wedding vows were made and celebrated in front of one's family, friends, work associates, and minister. To go outside the bounds of the relationship with the abuse is to renege on the sacred rite of marriage, the "promise" made to the greater community.

The mere thought of reporting abuse may elicit fears of retaliatory violence, death, harm to the children, and the general fear of the unknown. Some victims feel that their relationship has been so bad for such a long time, that they have come to accept it as "normal" and they are "beaten down." The consequent depressive and lethargic mental state makes reaching out for help seem too burdensome a task.

Though reporting abuse is a major hurdle to overcome for both women and men, it is inevitable that "thoughts" of reporting are also accompanied by wonderings about the consequent, hypothesized future. Once all the "pieces land," most always, the primary concern for both parents is their relationship with the children. Men and women fear that a major "shake-up" of their family poses the risk of losing access to or custody of their children. The threat of loss of custody is often presented to the victim as part of the abuse. Both women and men may not report abuse due to feeling overwhelmed at the prospect of raising children alone. Some victims cannot bear the feeling that they failed to keep their family together.

Obstacles Specific to Men Reporting Abuse

Several studies indicate that men are less likely than women to report abuse (Galdas, 2005; Cook 2009). There are both internal and external obstacles for men to report. Internally or psychologically, men traumatized in childhood may lack the awareness of abuse occurring, as well as a lack of initiative to deal with the problem. Adult males exposed to aggression as children tend to become somewhat tolerant of future aggression perpetrated against them (Berkowitz, 1974). Van der Kolk (1986) discussed consequences of males traumatized in childhood and emphasized the intense dependency on their partner, accompanied by the development of a loss of personal initiative. Men with a PTSD diagnosis have been found to exhibit learned helplessness, along with the loss of a sense of control of their destiny (van der Kolk, 1986).

As children, males who are physically attacked have three obvious choices: 1) hitting back and being perceived as aggressive; 2) running away and appearing weak; and 3) minimizing pain and appearing strong in the eyes of peers. In adulthood, the choices presented are quite different. Male victims of domestic violence tend to take the third of option of minimizing the abuse, out of fear of being arrested or becoming an object of ridicule ("wimp") (Cook, 1997; Flynn, 1990; Fontes, 1998; George, 2003).

For the male victim of domestic abuse, his state of victimization and his PTSD symptoms render him at complete odds with the twin ideals of male conditioning: being strong and in control. Conditioning short-circuits creative thinking, forces suppression of vulnerability and denial of hurtful feelings, and ultimately results in avoidance of the "victim" label at all costs. In the context of patriarchy, being a male victim is an inherent contradiction (Ghanim, 2012). An independent man is supposed to deal with problems that arise on his own. Reporting abuse is asking for help and would make him less of a man. Studies show that when injuries are severe, men are not just likely to not report assaults by women, but also are reluctant to report assault by other men (Hines, Malley-Morrision, 2005). Rather than face a diminishment of one's manhood, it is preferable to remain in denial that abuse has occurred. Throughout history, a man who is physically and emotionally abused by a woman - a man literally and figuratively beaten by a woman - is recognized as a loathsome creature.

Additionally, there are very real external obstacles for men that contemplate reporting abuse. Firstly, there is the societal bias that rigidly stereotypes women as victims and men as abusers. There is indeed a societal expectation that men will be more aggressive and violent than women (Lightdale and Prentice, 1994; Ghanim, 2012). A corollary to this is that abuse of men is not treated seriously and is often derided as a laughing matter. Consequently, many men believe that they won't be believed by law enforcement if they report abuse. Hamel (2005) discussed the bias within law enforcement to arrest males in cases of domestic violence. Hence, there is a real fear among men that even when they are the reporting party, they will be falsely arrested when police arrive on the scene. In summarizing the results of a study, Linda Mills (2008) reported that: "Despite the significant increase we've seen in the arrests of women in the past decade, police are still much more likely to take a report and make an arrest if the victim is a woman." (p. 35).

When men do seek help in domestic violence situations, there has been a glaring lack of resources and support services until very recently. Douglas and Hines (2011) conducted the first-ever large-scale national survey of men who sought help for heterosexual intimate partner violence. Their study included the finding that between half and two-thirds of male victims who sought help from police, DV hotlines, or DV agencies were told in one form or another that "we only help women." The study further revealed that in contrast to hotlines and law enforcement, men's concerns were taken seriously by 68% of mental health professionals, but only 30% offered useful information. In addition to professional clinicians, men reported that the best sources for help were friends, neighbors, relatives, lawyers, and ministers.

Obstacles for Victims to Leave Abusive Relationships

There are more commonalities than differences for why men and women stay and endure abusive relationships. For most parents where abuse is part of the relationship, children are the major priority. Some victims stay in the family home so that they can protect their children from the abusive partner. It is documented that abusive wives are as likely to exhibit violence toward children as abusive husbands (Straus & Smith, 1990; Margolin & Gordis, 2003). There also exist concerns of losing custody, having to raise children as a single parent, or suffering a decrease in living standards for themselves and children. Of course, when violence is severe, there are genuine fears of children being harmed or killed.

Over time, many victims feel too depressed and hopeless to initiate any assertive actions. They may lack knowledge of available resources and believe there is nowhere safe to go. Some think of themselves as a failure if they cannot make their marriage "work." For some victims, their religious beliefs have them firmly convinced that they will never leave under any circumstances.

Due to the controlling behaviors of their partner or due to their own shame about their situation, some victims become isolated and lack the support needed to help plan an escape. The thought of leaving the relationship may bring fears of retaliation, stalking, or being killed by their partner. Despite years of hostile arguments, frightening silences, and tense uncertainties, some women or men are still very much caught in the illusion of romantic love, feel deeply for their spouse, and believe that they have an "inner goodness" or a "good heart." The wish to "rediscover" that good heart transforms one's sane instinct for self-protection from a dangerous person into an irrational desire to provide whatever is necessary to revive the goodness underneath the bad behavior. In this case, they rationalize and make excuses for the abuse, and develop the belief that if they are a "good enough" spouse, then their partner will change.

The issue of the unique attachment that a couple forms is not given adequate attention, which further isolates the victim who does attempt to reach out and then experiences a lack of understanding. Just as each person is unique, so too each couple shares a bond that is fully unique to them and often unfathomable to outsiders. The most significant advance in the study of psychology since the instinctual theory posited by Freud is the discovery that it is imperative that human beings attach to others. When the intimacy of committed, long-term partnership is added to the equation, the obvious associations of romance, love, family, children, and sex serve to strengthen the bonds of attachment. The need for attachment becomes such a powerful motivating force in the psyche that it supersedes moral judgments that outsiders have about goodness or badness, health or dysfunction, equality or abuse. To help victims awaken and leave abusive relationships, we must first join their predicament by understanding the uniqueness of their relationship and their life-and-death need for attachment.

Obstacles Specific to Men to Leave Abusive Relationships

Men are socialized to be responsible and competent, which includes commitment to marriage (Hines & Malley-Morisson, 2001). It is universally established that with commitment, comes the responsibility to provide for and protect their family. Despite the tendency for some males to abdicate responsibility and fidelity, leaving the family is often accompanied by the feeling that you are "less than a man" (Cook, 1997). For some, along with commitment to family, their basic integrity is on the line. There exists the common male ethos of: "You are only as good as your word." That word is represented by the public commitment made to one's partner, family, friends, and community and is violated at a cost to one's identity.

There is a cognitive dissonance with regard to viewing oneself – a member of the more aggressive and violent gender – as a victim of a woman's aggression and violence. It is doubly dissonant that a male victim may fear retribution for leaving. This retaliation may take the form of stalking, the spread of malicious rumors to family, friends, and coworkers, and even false accusations of domestic violence. Also, there is typically greater concern for men than women about loss of contact or custody of children.

As with female victims, many male victims have experienced abuse and violence in their family of origin.

These dysfunctional models of relationship have been internalized in childhood and are reenacted in adulthood. Many men and women are caught in a lifelong cycle of abuse, whereby violence is perpetrated, distance between the couple occurs, followed by the honeymoon stage filled with affections, apologies, and promises to get help. The impulses to commit acts of violence are now replaced by impulses to regain the seemingly lost relationship. The subsequent make up dinners, make up flowers, and make up sex do not in any way achieve the necessary thoughtful decisions and considered steps that could possibly heal the broken relationship.

Maternal instinct is well established in our culture as a feminine quality. A corollary of this instinct is the scenario of a woman rescuing or saving her partner from drugs, danger, or depravity of one form or another. However, there seems to be a definite discounting of the qualities of nurturance and compassion that many men possess. The caring nature of a man may manifest in desires and efforts to improve the life of his partner, protect her from physical harm, help her be free of a struggle to make ends meet, or rescue her from a bad situation with her family or even her previous relationship. As with women, the male counterpart to this rescuing dynamic often persists after the loving relationship is over. For both men and women victimized by abuse, there is a strong tendency to view their partner as a really good person rather than as a dangerous person from which to flee. So, women and men stay.

Another motivating factor is analogous in a lighter way with the Las Vegas gambler who stays too long at the table. You have invested your time, money, energy, and with your continued presence at the table, you feel the strong pull of the game. For those losing at cards and for those losing in an abusive relationship, hope does spring eternal. Sooner or later, the cards will turn in your favor. Sooner or later, the relationship with your partner will return to those joyous, adventurous days of first meeting, first making a connection, first sharing a laugh, and eyes first meeting with the silent acknowledgement of love. So, you stubbornly stay at the poker table, you stubbornly stay in the abusive relationship.

It appears to be human nature to engage in the pursuit of recapturing, irrespective of the merits of our efforts. The attempt to recapture an earlier moment in life can be the basis for accomplishment - reliving the unbridled joy you experienced when you showed off the toy blocks you put together as a toddler. You may recall the big smiles, hugs, joys, and love that came your way. People sometimes try to recapture the "high" moment when they first consumed a tasty sweet treat, or first felt the relaxing effects of a pill, or first sniffed a line of cocaine. So, recapturing can also be a basis for addictions. Hence, the saying: "you are always chasing that first high." Recapturing can play a powerful role in staying too long at the card table, as well as staying too long in the abusive relationship.

Recommendations for Battered Men

Safety Plan (Immediate):

1. Never retaliate (violence is violence, no matter who started it; retaliation is wrong and you will be arrested).
2. Be aware of triggers for angry responses for both your partner and yourself.
3. Leave if possible.
4. Keep essential items close at hand to leave at moment's notice (driver's license, cell phone, passport, cash, credit cards, checkbook, etc.).
5. Log all abusive actions (dates, times, places, events, witnesses).
6. Document injuries (cuts, bruises, scratches, etc.).
7. Photos of injuries.
8. Record / videotape incidents of abuse.
9. Keep information outside the home (with trusted friend).
10. Report violent incidents to police (get copy of police report).
11. Report injuries (medical personnel unlikely to inquire if a man is victim of abuse).
12. Seek advice from certified domestic violence program (restraining orders, temporary custody of children, legal aid).

Keep in Mind:

1. You are not alone as a male victim of abuse.
2. Without outside intervention, abuse in relationships tends to increase in frequency and intensity over time.
3. Police departments receive training on both male and female batterers.

4. Police do have the obligation to protect men and their children.
5. Domestic violence shelters to help men do exist.

Questions to Contemplate:

1. How should power between partners be divided in relationships?
2. Is your relationship healthy, functional, dysfunctional, abusive?
3. Are you comfortable being yourself in the relationship?
4. Do you have concerns or fears about your partner's anger?
5. Do you believe that you have good control over your own anger?
6. Do you need outside intervention to cope with your relationship?
7. Are there steps you can take before you call the police?
8. Does the "legal system" treat men and women equally?
9. Should the "system" treat men and women equally?
10. Do you naturally "favor" men or women?
11. What attitudes do you have that are "sexist"?
12. What is your definition of a 21st century "man"?

Recommendations for Clinicians

The first order of business for a clinician to be of real help to a victim of domestic violence is to form a connection and build a bond based on trust and a caring interest in them. At the same time, you must possess stability as a person and genuine confidence in your own competence. The work of domestic violence treatment is too crucial and too immediate to do with anything less than knowledge of resources and experience working with victims and perpetrators. Eye contact is essential, and the eyes are usually your first instrument to communicate that you know what you are doing.

One of the most frustrating, and completely out-of-touch things someone could say to a person in an abusive relationship is to "just leave him," or "just leave her." As a clinician working with people involved in domestic violence, the last thing I will say to an abused person is "just leave." The one crucial exception to that is if the patient, the children, or even the perpetrator is in immediate danger. If you sense through the dialogue or with the intuition from experience that someone will likely either perpetrate or be the victim of physical violence, then you must intervene. You must take steps to promptly initiate – with urgency – the process of obtaining the needed outside assistance to ensure non-violence and peace.

In the absence of "red flags" of immediate danger, it is incumbent on the clinician to realize that the victim has not only heard "just leave" from others, but they have also said, "just leave" to themselves 150 times. Obviously, there is greater complexity to what is first presented by the patient in this situation. Women have their own particular real and valid reasons to stay in an abusive relationship, as do men. To truly be of help, the clinician must empathize with the needs and feelings of the patient and communicate that empathy either verbally or non-verbally. You must have the flexibility to communicate empathy and understanding either subtly or more overtly. You are "reading" your patient to determine which approach is required of you. You are in service.

This exchange of the patient's needs and feelings with your return empathic response – on the level required – is an absolute prerequisite to help facilitate any escape from abuse. You have to learn about the person in front of you as a unique human being. Additionally, this unique person you are trying to help has a unique and "special" relationship with their abuser that you need to fully comprehend. To that end, I usually begin the process by finding out what is so special about their partner and what is so special about their relationship. When I am at my best, my initial stance is one of genuine curiosity and lack of judgment. It is a stance grounded in an ethos that is both caring and professional.

Clinicians must take great care not to retraumatize the patient with their words or tone of voice. No matter how well-meaning you may feel, the "just leave" proclamation is a judgment and may be experienced as an intrusive command, another violation of boundaries, or a retraumatization of abuse. It is neither caring nor professional.

An overall goal of treatment is to maintain a balance between respecting personal boundaries and guarding against intrusiveness on the one hand, and at the same time, facilitating the patient's exploration of their psyches, their priorities, and ultimately their course of action. Things work best when the "breakthrough ideas" come from the patient. When the very idea of leaving the relationship comes up, the obstacles to carrying that out must first be explored. Obstacles involve practicalities, emotions, and attachments.

Before victims come to seek your help, they have likely already talked with close confidantes. In this stressful and frightening situation, you must provide what few others can:

1. A keen knowledge of dynamics of domestic violence.
2. Wisdom grounded in experience.
3. A big heart rooted in your personal motivation to be of help and service to others.

Recommendations for Society

Domestic violence is a problem for people, not just women. In "The Unfair Sex" (1995), Wendy McElroy stated: ". . . injustice is the inevitable result of treating men as a separate and antagonistic class, rather than as individuals who share the same humanity as women. Men are not monsters. They are our fathers, brothers, sons, husbands, and lovers. They should not be made to stand before a legal system that presumes their guilt." Hines and Malley-Morrison (2005) asserted the traditional ethos of Native Americans that: ". . . to eliminate family violence (or violence in general) both types of aggression must be addressed, and the common practice in the majority judicial system of blaming the male for the conflict and ignoring the women's role is inappropriate and ineffective" (pp. 44-45).

As previously mentioned, until very recently there has been a glaring lack of support services for men. In addition, there exist other underserved populations including the elderly, same-sex couples, and transgendered people (Mills, 2008; Douglas and Hines, 2011). Though male victims try different approaches when seeking help and attempt to use a variety of resources, for the most part their experiences tend to be more negative than positive. When men or women in this depressed situation reach out for help and are rebuffed, their overall mental health status is compromised.

When it comes to understanding male perspectives on domestic violence, the bias against men as victims is real. A primary root of this lack of understanding is society's traditional punitive position toward perpetrators, as opposed to approaches involving understanding, empathy, and education. As discussed above, men may well act with more aggression than women, and so there exists a glaring need to provide males – especially young males – with tools and outlets for their aggressive tendencies. The need to establish programs that promote assertive tools and healthy, creative outlets for men is urgent, as evidenced by the worldwide, overwhelming, unrelenting, daily assaults on the physical body and life itself.

Specifically, here are some recommendations for further discussion and analysis to deal with the problem of domestic violence in our society:

1. Gender inclusive public education concerning domestic violence, along with outreach materials for potential victims (Hines and Douglas, 2011).
2. College and secondary school curricula in the social sciences designed to prepare future mental health and social service practitioners about common experiences of all victims, regardless of victim and perpetrator gender
3. Increase in training about culture and gender diversity for clinicians who provide services for victims of domestic violence.
4. Re-evaluation by police departments with regard to how to handle domestic violence incidents and how to respond when victims do not meet gendered stereotypes.
5. Legal assistance that is more readily available, more affordable, and better trained in domestic violence.
6. Thorough screening of all clients and patients for abusive experiences, with ready availability of information on getting help for domestic violence.
7. Focused research examining the effectiveness of public education, screenings, trainings, and treatment techniques in the field of domestic violence.
8. Focused research on domestic violence that is inclusive of both genders, with regard to related mental health issues, drug and alcohol addictions, abuse in childhood, school problems, bullying, and truancy, etc.
9. Focused research on the multilevel effects of domestic violence on children regarding their physical, cognitive, emotional, and relational development, and school performance.
10. Coordination of methods and goals of domestic violence treatment providers, shelter workers, police

departments, child service workers, and the legal system.

Patriarchy Reigns

On the level of the individual, men predominantly possess greater stature, strength, weight, athleticism, and experience in hand-to-hand combat than women do. On the macro level of the overall ethos of society, patriarchy has ruled the day. Throughout history, with few exceptions, society has been governmentally ruled, financially controlled, and historically chronicled by men. It is inarguable that societies have been patriarchal in nature. Simplistically viewed, it may follow that hunting is considered to be more valuable than gathering, whether in the time of the Neanderthal, homo erectus, or the present-day time of modern humans. Women in ancient times tending to the nascent nests and caves may well have been subordinate to their male counterparts who used the physical prowess and "authority" needed to deal with predators and prey to dominate their female partners as well. Allowing for exceptions, this patriarchal dynamic may play out with women of modern times taking care of child-rearing and homemaking. While the modern man leaves home each day to work in fields, factories, and offices, and uses power and authority to both earn the keep of his family and dominate his female partner.

Another primitive phenomenon with a modern-day analogue involves the violence perpetrated by men against women who are pregnant or of child-bearing age. The male instinct to propagate genes may well inspire the strongest urges to control, keep in line, and fully dominate a pregnant woman who is "showing" or a woman of appropriate age for childbirth. Recent data reveals that women of child-bearing ages are at greatest risk of physical violence at the hands of their partner. Ages 20 to 24 present the greatest risk of violence, with ages 35 to 49 at the next greatest risk, with the least risk occurring for women ages 50 and above. Domestic violence during pregnancy remains a significant problem worldwide and is associated with adverse outcomes for newborns. Obvious consequences include internal bleeding, damage to the fetus, low birth weight, preterm births, miscarriage, depression and poor self-care. In the United States, prenatal providers do not routinely screen for domestic violence (Bailey, 2010). Male perpetration against vulnerable, child-bearing women receives little attention, yet it represents another method of male dominance in society.

Perhaps, the most under discussed and potentially controversial topic of all has to do with the automatic, non-conscious attribution of masculinity to the deity. For those who possess belief in God, would not God with status and power much beyond human form, exist beyond gender? Yet, seemingly without thought or wonderment, God is virtually always referred to with the masculine pronoun. It seems to me that at the birth of all religions, it was men who served as the elders, the elite, the powerful, the members of the ruling councils, and significantly, the chroniclers of the words of religious prophets. So once multifarious Gods were subsumed by monotheism, God was forever given a male identity

According to Ghanim (2012), "...monotheistic religion has helped strengthen the patriarchal context that supports domination and control of women," (p. 57). The hold on the seat of power for the masculine God may be subtle, but the consequences are both pervasive in the world and persistent throughout all historical eras. Though this appears to be a firmly sealed, taboo subject for exploration, an investigation and discussion of the masculine God ethos would prove to be quite stimulating and fruitful to bring both a fresh, modern re-balancing of the genders and a sorely needed cooperative spirit to women and men.

It is my belief that males who suffer violence at the hands of women can be more fully addressed and cared for if and when our society comes to terms with patriarchy in all its forms. Perhaps then, a long overdue balancing of the genders can occur. A further "perhaps" may involve the creation of a world with less violence and greater harmony.

The "Good Man"

As a counterweight to patriarchal society, there exist multitudes of men attempting to live their lives genuinely striving to be a "responsible man" and a "good man." Most typically, these valiant men – in every sense of the word – are overshadowed by the often sensationalized, dramatized, and even exalted "bad man" or "bad boy." There are many men who have internalized in childhood a non-violence way of being from their mother or father, or have developed their own strong, predisposition against ever using their physicality to perpetrate against a woman, or any vulnerable person. This ethos can be so strong and resolute that they refrain from physical contact even when they are being attacked by their female partner. Typically, these unsung males possess a fierce loyalty toward their family and are willing to tolerate abuse, stay with their partner, and continue to work to improve their relationship and themselves. Let's not take for granted what some would say is the expected way for men to behave, and instead promote, celebrate, and give at least equal attention to the "good man."

Healing the Rift

The focus in this chapter has been on intimate partner violence, with particular attention given to male victims. However, to fully contemplate and address the problem of domestic violence for men and women, we must pull back the lens and objectively analyze and understand the overall dimensions of the problem. Thus, it is crucial that the issue be considered beyond the immediate incident, beyond the most recent statistics, and beyond anecdotal accounts of "war" between the genders. As a clinician, theoretician, and activist for most of my career, I have primarily discussed the issues in the "female camp" and debated the issues in the "male camp." Researching and writing this chapter has helped me to gain a broader perspective and come to the realization that the "camps" are too far apart in their attitudes and approaches to the problem. What is required of these "camps" parallels what is basically required for any healthy, egalitarian adult relationship: Women and men must engage in formalized dialogues which include the willingness to cooperate, open mindedness, genuine inquiry, listening, understanding, empathy, and the brainstorming and exchange of ideas that lead to coordinated actions to both reduce domestic violence and promote interactions of mutuality and peace.

References

Andersen, T. (2013). Against the wind: Male victimization and the ideal of manliness. *Journal of Social Work,* Vol. 13, (3), pp. 231-247.

Archer, J. (2000). Sex differences in aggression between heterosexual partners: A meta-analytic review. *Psychological Bulletin, 126* (5), pp. 651-680.

Bailey, B. (2010). Partner violence during pregnancy: Prevalence, effects, screening, and management. *International Journal of Women's Health,* Vol. 2, pp. 183-197.

Berkowitz, E. (1974). Some determinants of impulsive aggression. *Psychological Review, 81:* pp. 165-176.

Bettencourt, B. and Miller, N. (1996). Gender differences in aggression as a function of provocation: A meta-analysis. *Psychological Bulletin,* Vol. 119 (3), pp. 422-447.

Braudy, L. (2003). From chivalry to terrorism: War and the changing nature of masculinity. New York: Alfred A. Knopf.

Centers for Disease Control and Prevention (2014). *The National Intimate Partner and Sexual Violence Survey,* https://www.cdc.gov/violenceprevention/nisvs/index.htm

Cho, H. (2012). Examining gender differences in the nature and context of intimate partner violence. *Journal of Interpersonal Violence,* Vol. 27, (13), pp. 2665-2684.

Cook, P. (2009). Abused Men: The hidden side of domestic violence: Westport, CT: Praeger.

Diamond, J. (1999). *Guns, germs, and steel: The fates of human societies.* New York: W.W. Norton & Company.

Douglas, E. and Hines, D. (2011). The help-seeking experiences of men who sustain intimate partner violence: An overlooked population and its implications for practice. *Journal of Family Violence,* Vol. 26, (6), pp. 473-485.

Finkelhor, D, Gelles, R., Hotaling, G., and Straus, M. (1983). *The dark side of families: Current family violence research.* Los Angeles: Sage Publications.

Ghanim, D. (2012). Gender violence: Theoretical overview. *In Violence and abuse in society.* Oxford, England: Praeger.

Hamel, J. (2014). Gender inclusive treatment of intimate partner abuse: Evidence-based approaches. New York: Springer Publishing Company.

Hines, D. and Malley-Morrision, K, (2005). Family violence in the United States. Los Angeles: Sage Publications.

Hoff, B. H. (2012, February 12). CDC Study: More men than women victims of intimate partner physical violence, psychological aggression. Retrieved from Stop Abusive and Violent Environments:

http://www.saveservices.org/2012/02/cdc-study-more-men-than-women-victims-of-partner-abuse/

Hyunkag, H. (2012). Examining gender differences in nature and context of intimate partner violence. *Journal of Interpersonal Violence,* Vol. 27, (13), pp. 2665-2684.

Ingalhalikar, M, et. al. (2014). Sex differences in the structural connectome of the human brain. Proceeding of the National Academy of Sciences of the United States of America, Vol. 111, (2), pp. 2665-2684.

Johnson, M. (2006). Control and conflict: gender symmetry and asymmetry in domestic violence. *Violence Against Women*, Vol. 12, (11), pp. 1003-1018.

Kimmel, M. (2017). Angry white men: American masculinity at the end of an era. New York: Nation Books.

Kret, M. and DeGelder, B. (2012). Reviews and perspectives: A review of sex differences in processing emotional signals. *Neuropsychologia Journal*, The Netherlands, Vol. 50, pp. 1211-1221.

Leslie, D. and Cavanough, M. (2005). *Current controversies on family violence*. Thousand Oaks, CA: Sage Publications.

Lightdale, J. and Prentice, D. (1994). Rethinking sex differences in aggression: aggressive behavior in the absence of social roles. *Personality and Social Psychology Bulletin*, Vol. 20, (1), pp. 34-44.

Lurito, J. (2001). Temporal lobe activation demonstrates sex-based differences during passive listening. *Neuroradiology*, Vol. 220, (1).

Marin, A. and Russo, N. (1999). Feminist perspectives on male violence against women in *What Causes Men's Violence Against Women*. Thousand Oaks, CA: Sage Publications, Inc.

McElroy, W. (1996). The unfair sex in Bender, D. et. al. *Family violence: Current controversies*. San Diego: Greenhaven Press, Inc.

Mills, L. (2008). Violent Partners: A breakthrough plan for ending the cycle of abuse. New York: Basic Books.

Mizen, R. and Morris, M. (2007). *On aggression and violence: An analytic perspective.* New York: Palgrave Macmillan.

Nettle, D. (2007). Empathizing and systematizing: What are they and what do they contribute to our understanding of psychological sex differences. *British Journal of Psychology,* Vol. 98, (2), pp. 237-255.

New York State Office for the Prevention of Domestic Violence (2017). Website: http://opdv.ny.gov/faqs/index.html#maleandfemale perps.

Pollack, W. (1998). *Real boys: Rescuing our sons from the myths of boyhood.* New York: Henry Holt and Company, LLC.

Straus, M. (1988). *Abuse and victimization across the lifespan.* Baltimore: Johns Hopkins University Press.

Van der Kolk, B. (1986). *The psychology of the trauma response. Psychological trauma.* Washington, D.C.: American Psychiatric Association Press.

Chapter 20 Summary

Relational Effects of Male Trauma

Society puts forth the idea that the mind and body are separate entities. This idea, which is universally accepted as mainstream, is false and does us all a disservice. The mind and body interact constantly. They are interconnected and interwoven; their sum makes the whole of who we are as people.

Our behavior, specifically how we react to situations, is a direct result of the mind-body connection. These perceptions have been developed over the course of our entire lives. It is shaped by every experience we have. Every joyful, disappointing, or traumatizing moment is stored in our unconscious mind. Our behavior is a reflection of those moments.

Dr. Joshua D. Wyner puts forth this fact in detail, followed by an explanation of the decision-making process as it relates to the mind-body connection. He says we are emotional beings first, then rational ones. Our emotions are first in line to analyze a situation. Then our rational mind jumps in.

In my experience, tense situations with Robert that resulted in angry outbursts were the result of allowing my emotions to grab hold of the wheel and decide where we go next. The awakening I had, described in the chapter on anger, occurred by allowing my rational mind to have a say in these matters as well.

The rational side contains my compassion, empathy, and patience. The emotional side is impulsive and reactionary. Rather than allowing my emotional perceptions to shape my response, I let those perceptions pass through into the rational stage as well. Then I paused and slowed down the situation to avoid acting out from a place of defensiveness and anger.

Once I did this, my reactions to Robert's mood swings were calm, patient, and composed – more often than not. Not only did my relationship benefit, but my serenity did as well.

From the perspective of a male survivor, many situations and interactions never pass from the emotional realm to the rational one. They perceive something as triggering, and unconsciously, the "primitive" mind kicks in. Their emotional, "primitive" brain is telling them that they need to protect themselves from a threat. That is why your spouse's behavior may be erratic and irrational at times. He is acting out from a place of trauma.

For any person, and to a greater degree with trauma survivors, the primitive brain acts independently from rational thought. It is a response to a perceived threat. Once the threat is gone, the brain returns to baseline functioning. When Robert and I escalate a discussion to a point of tension, I have found it is important for me to disengage and step away. It allows both of us to cool down. We can address the issue later when it can be discussed rationally.

These patterns of thinking and reacting can be changed. Dr. Wyner lays out several techniques that can help a male survivor change his thinking. Exposure therapy can help a male survivor become comfortable with intimacy. Mindfulness, meditation, and breathing techniques help to slow down the pattern of thought. This allows space for thoughtful, rational responses.

Everyone is guilty of acting out emotionally and irrationally at times. It is part of the human experience. For me, identifying it, and taking steps to slow down my thinking made a big difference in interacting with Robert. For male survivors, treatment is available that can change the patterns of thinking that trauma has created.

Chapter 20

Relational Effects of Male Trauma

Joshua D. Wyner, Ph.D.
Interim Associate Chair
Marriage & Family Therapy Program
The Chicago School of Professional Psychology

One of the most persistent and inaccurate myths still pervading our society is our continued misunderstanding (and oversimplification) of the mind-body relationship. From an early age, we are typically taught that these are separate entities; that while they interact, they are also wholly distinct. The problem here is that this model misses the truth behind a truly dual relationship: mind and body are each a feature of who we are. To paraphrase the great neuroscientist Dan Siegel, the self (consciousness) is like the shore – where does the sand end and the water begin? Instead, we talk about how the two aspects of the shore (water and sand) interact. When our bodies are stressed, the emotional self is too. When the self is calm, so is the body.

The rational (slow and thoughtful) and emotional (fast and automatic) are similarly misunderstood as distinct, rather than entities which intertwine to create the whole self. Instead, they are more accurately understood as a dyad, interacting and communicating with each other to create action. In order to understand how we make choices and engage with the world around us, we must understand these systems and dualistic relationships. For it is only through understanding them that we can begin to understand the complex dance of trauma and how those who experience it engage with their world.

The Neurobiology of Trauma

A Systemic View of Decision-Making

To understand our response to trauma, we must first explore the delicate balance of cognition and emotion in decision-making. Although we often like to think of ourselves as rational creatures suffering from the curse of primitive emotions, the reality is that we are emotional creatures first and rational ones second. For some, this idea is terrifying, and the natural inclination is to respond defensively: "This isn't true for me! I'm rational!" (in a strong, emotionally charged tone). This truth, though, is what allows us to function and enjoy our daily lives. Our emotions serve as our first pass *heuristic* system (something that processes information very quickly using shortcuts). They examine the environment in the moment, using all of the senses at once, and come to an immediate conclusion about which options are safest. These emotionally acceptable options are then presented to the rational self for final selection. To put it another way, our emotions do the initial work in sorting our environment, and then our rational selves help organize those responses in order to make sense of the world and act!

Memory & Emotions

In addition to this decision-making role, our brains also utilize these emotional heuristics to distinguish important events from unimportant ones when determining which things to remember and which to forget. When you enter a room, most of the environment is emotionally empty (for example, we tend to have no feelings about the neutral white walls or carpet). Instead, a few key items will typically stand out – perhaps a friend you were coming to meet, or the projector screen for an upcoming presentation. This filtering of our environment is necessary to avoid overload: just imagine if you had to stop and consider the color and shape of every object in a room before you could proceed! Instead, important events are "tagged" with the strong emotion, which in turn lets the brain identify them as memorable.

Trauma and Decision-Making

When we experience severe trauma, our bodies respond as they would to any severe threat: trying to survive by any means necessary. The perceived threat is "tagged" by the emotional system as important and vital so much so that our cognition is rendered virtually useless. There is now only one choice available: address the imminent threat. Instead of accessing our full rational selves, the cognitive processes are "tuned down" by the powerful emotion. The prefrontal cortex (one of the key brain regions responsible for turning our cognitions and emotions into action) is downregulated, allowing the fast, emotional heuristics to take over and mobilize us without the cumbersome interference of slow, rational thoughts. At the same time, the sympathetic nervous system is *upregulated* in order to let our bodies actually move away from the threat (this is the same system that is turned up when we do exercise, feel panic, or take stimulants).

Take, for example, the classic example of a person walking through a forest and encountering a bear. For most, the immediate emotional processing of this experience would present only one or two options to the rational self: run or hide. That's it. And that's good. If this didn't happen, the rational self would be allowed to sit and slowly examine the environment. In the time it might take to sit and ponder the bear, the individual would already be eaten! So instead, the emotional system turns down the cognitive functions of the brain in order to let the reflexive, emotional system take over and move the person to safety. Once the threat is gone, the brain returns to its default state, where our cognitive and emotional systems are once again in balance.

Memory and Decision-Making

A consequence of this experience, though, is that this traumatic event has been tagged with a strong (typically unpleasant) emotion. By doing so, we've also primed the brain to consider it important enough to remember. In some ways, this is adaptive: something dangerous happened, and we want to make sure we recognize similar dangers in the future so we can avoid them. Unfortunately, this also leads to an increased chance of recalling the event when similar, but different events occur.

The result? Post-traumatic effects. Imagine again the person who encountered that bear. Back in the safety of the city, they step outside only to hear a friend step on a twig. This sound primes the now strong memory of the bear attack, immediately retrieving that memory, which included a ramping up of their sympathetic nervous system (fight and/or flight) and the down regulation of cognitive function. In short, they are now suddenly thrust back into that moment, unable to think as clearly, and ready to combat the danger of a bear. Of course, this time there is no bear, but they are unable to fully realize this and respond appropriately.

The Relational Effects of Trauma

Within the context of a relationship, this recall of trauma can become even more significant. To recall a memory, we need only to relive a small piece of the whole – perhaps a smell, sound, or visual cue. For better and worse, relationships are overflowing with emotional cues, above and beyond the daily sensory ones. This combination of sensory and emotional cues greatly increases the chance of triggering one of those traumatic memories, in particular if the trauma is a relational one such as rape or domestic violence. Imagine if, instead of a bear, we now consider someone who was sexually molested as a child. In addition to any sounds or images, they may be (and often are) triggered by a partner's touch, breath, or even smell. Entering a bedroom or even being alone with a partner could be enough to trigger the memory and return them to that reflexive "fight or flight" state.

How to Move Forward

Fortunately, the flip side of this intimate connection between experience and memory is that new memory patterns can be formed over time, and the depth of emotional connection with a safe loved one can have a similar emotional strength to those initial memories. These *corrective experiences* can serve to counteract the traumatic one, returning function to the traumatized individual. Specifically, they can relearn associations between specific sensations and memories, replacing the trauma with something more innocuous and even pleasant.

In cases of sexual trauma, for example, we may use exposure therapy techniques to associate nudity and touch with intimate connection rather than coerced sexuality. One of the most well-known examples of this process is Sensate Focus, first developed by Masters and Johnson[1]. This process combines exposure therapy with mindfulness approaches – it recognizes the innate need for touch in humans, while also acknowledging the maladaptive relationship with touch that the trauma victim might have.

Under this model, couples acknowledge the need for touch as well as the negative expectations and beliefs the trauma victim might have regarding being touched (for example, any touch might lead to sexual activity, even when wanted). The individuals must therefore relearn the value of physical touch in and of itself, without the inherent association with sex and arousal. One example of a Sensate

Focus technique is "skin time," wherein a couple managing sexual trauma is asked by the therapist to temporarily refrain from intercourse or any other uncomfortable sexual activity. They are then tasked with a nightly ritual of skin-to-skin contact, often beginning with hand holding and slowly working up to full-body nude contact over the course of weeks and months. Each week, the therapist meets with the couple to evaluate their experiences and reactions, carefully increasing the timing and level of nudity based upon the traumatized individual's comfort level. The goal is for the activity to be mildly uncomfortable, but not traumatic – it should not trigger a sympathetic (panicky) state. As this becomes more and more comfortable, the timing and level of nudity are increased, until the couple is comfortable being naked together.

Another related approach for managing trauma is the use of mindfulness to manage one's sympathetic responses. Unlike Sensate Focus, mindfulness techniques may be done individually. The simplest example is some form of mindful meditation. Unlike Eastern meditations which focus on emptying the mind, mindfulness meditations recognize that the individual may have thoughts and feelings during the process, and instead help the patient respond to them with a less powerful physical response. The individual is taught to manage their breathing by taking a breath over four seconds, waiting four seconds, exhaling for four seconds, and then waiting four seconds again before repeating. As uncomfortable thoughts and feelings arise, they are instructed to simply acknowledge them as they continue to breathe. The breathing prevents the body from entering a panic state, which allows the individual to experience those uncomfortable thoughts decoupled from the usual responses that come with it. Over time, they learn to tolerate the difficult thoughts and feelings.

A final example of trauma work is a treatment modality known as Dialectical Behavior Therapy (DBT). This form of therapy uses similar principles to those described earlier (including mindfulness, self-soothing, and exposure) while also recognizing the importance of acceptance. In DBT, a non-judgmental environment is key, filled with positive regard and understanding. Rather than using words like "bad" or "unfair," DBT simply describes events as they are. "I react badly," might become "My heart rate increases," or "I begin to sweat more." The client is taught "radical acceptance" – a stance that emphasizes accepting reality rather than fighting it merely because it might be unpleasant. Instead of pushing back, they are instructed to explore the uncomfortable feelings more fully, using anything available (e.g. meditation, music, touch, food, sleep, or exercise) to instead tolerate the feelings without becoming overwhelmed.

Virtually every approach to trauma begins from an understanding that the individual is not in control of their response: through their trauma, they have learned an automatic but dysfunctional way of responding to certain events. The only way out is to acknowledge these responses and learn new, healthier ones through the highly effective process of controlled exposure. With patience and proper guidance, any painful memory can be managed and overcome.

References

Weiner, Linda; Avery-Clark, Constance (2017). *Sensate Focus in Sex Therapy: The Illustrated Manual.* New York: Routledge.

Chapter 21 Summary

Multicultural Issues Related to
Male Abuse Survivors

The culture we grow up in will determine how we respond to the world. Culture is bigger than any one family and is connected an individual's societal context. Culture is beyond skin tone, but can also involve other factors such as geographical location, educational level, social economic status, being a single parent, and gender. Each of these factors can have an impact on one's worldview and how they interact with others.

How one's culture views abuse is varied. This chapter delves into the many ways in which different cultures establish taboo subjects and what is an "acceptable" response.

In my husband's home and culture, to admit that he was abused was not something that was easily accepted; in fact it was minimized at first by his mother. Their family culture was driven more by the model that strong men defend themselves, and if something happened, he must have wanted it.

The one aspect that appears consistently across all cultures is that men do not want to talk about being abused.

Chapter 21

Multicultural Issues Related to Male Abuse Survivors

Erin Langdon, M.A.
The Chicago School of Professional Psychology

There is a haunting question about the relationship between culture and sexual violence, how it is perceived by dominant groups towards populations of color, or how minorities themselves view the abuse. The perceptions shape reactions (both survivor and protector), if and whether there is prosecution of the accused, and how the story of the abuse is accepted or perceived. At play is not only sexism, racism, and dominance, but the inequality of power and structure (McGuffey, 2013; Collins, 2004).

Our life development is part of an ecological system from birth to death (Gardiner, 2011). This system shapes our beliefs, our identity, our sexuality, and our understanding of shame, power, and seeking help. Thinking or thought processes are altered and distributed differently within and from culture to culture (Prado, Chadha, & Booth, 2011). When it comes to abuse, culture plays a very important role.

But culture is also a thought process evolved from traditions, myths, and experience.

There are many examples of how different cultures respond to abuse, and how culture affects people's responses to abuse victims and authorities. For example, an African American child is the victim of sexual abuse. The mother may decide not to contact the police. White Americans may ask "why not?" But, from an African American perspective, there is the "collectivist" belief that family business is taken care of within family, or the belief that law enforcement acts with brutality and callousness against people of color. A Cambodian family, either in the United States or Cambodia, may acquiesce to allowing authorities to remove their child from their home because of their previously disempowering experiences with law enforcement. The Hmong community also tends to be unsympathetic to victims of sexual abuse. They are not prepared to provide support or resources to affected children Hmong families typically hide problems that are culturally taboo. Their fear of shame overrules their acceptance of the incident (Xiong et. al., 2006). In countries like Saudi Arabia, there is denial of child sexual abuse. These examples show why an individual's culture must be taken into consideration in helping both the survivor and the family that surrounds them.

Regardless of national origin, there seems to be a near universal cultural ignorance regarding male sexual abuse. Societies have rules for man behavior and rites of passage to relieve men of any perceived femininity. Males are typically seen as warriors and do not experience emotional pain. In some countries, the belief is so powerful that it is beaten or raped into the consciousness of the boy as he grows. In the United States, from birth male children are told that "men don't cry," or it is girly to show emotions other than anger. Males are expected to be strong, not vulnerable, and to be the sexual aggressor. It takes little imagination to understand why a boy or a man will not report being sexually assaulted or abused. His entire manhood is put in question, not only by authorities who do not always believe them, but by family and friends who scoff at the idea he didn't willing participate. The cultural mindset must change in order to relieve the male victim of feeling victimized twice – once by the perpetrator and again by society.

References

Al Eissa, M., Almuneef, M. (2010). Child abuse and neglect in Saudi Arabia: Journey of recognition to implementation of national prevention strategies *Child Abuse Neglect, 34* (2010), pp. 28-33

Collins, R. 2004. *Ritual interaction chains.* Princeton: Princeton University Press.

Gardiner, H. W. (2011). *Living across Cultures: Cross cultural human development* (5th ed.). Boston: Pearson Education.

McGuffey, C. (2013). Rape and racial appraisals: Culture, intersectionality, and black women's accounts of sexual assault. *Du Bois Review: Social Science Research on Race, 10*(1), 109-130. doi:10.1017/S1742058X12000355

Prado, J., Chadha, A., & Booth, J. R. (2011, November 1). The brain network for deductive reasoning: A quantitative meta-analysis of 28 neuroimaging studies. *Journal of Cognitive Neuroscience, 23*(11), 3483-3497. http://dx.doi.org/10.1162/jocn_a_00063

Xiong, Z. B., Tuicomepee, A., LaBlanc, L., & Rainey, J. (2006). Hmong immigrants' perceptions of family secrets and recipients of disclosure. Families in Society: *The Journal of Contemporary Social Services, 87*(2), 231-239.

Chapter 22 Summary

Concerns about Parenting

In this chapter, my husband voices the fears and concerns of many survivors and their spouses about parenting, and lays out the constructive ways in which spouses can be supportive. He presents the theory that many of these fears are normal responses to the great responsibility of raising a child, but for survivors, there are additional layers of self-doubt, false assumptions by society, and in many cases a lack of good role models.

The silver lining in the pain that Robert experienced as he honestly and courageously faced his past, is the strength and hope that he demonstrates as father and role model for our son Lawrence, and for the many men that his truth will help.

Chapter 22

Concerns about Parenting

Robert A. Carey, Psy.D.
County of San Bernardino, California
Dept. of Mental Health

Fredrick Douglass said, "It is easier to build strong children than to repair broken men."

Male survivors are not exactly broken men, but we carry scars that no one else can see. Scars that have built up over the years to form a protective armor but oftentimes interfere with forming close relationships. So how then, do we help to build strong children when we become fathers? And what can you as the spouse do to help?

Parenting is an intensely vulnerable experience. Your child's smile can make you feel like the most important person alive, but sometimes one tear can crush you into almost nothing. Embracing vulnerability can be difficult for anyone, but men in general, and male survivors specifically, often face unique challenges opening up and exposing ourselves emotionally.

As men we're taught to be strong, independent, and determined. We're encouraged to look at every activity as a competition and every competition as a test of our worth.

Vulnerability is weakness; weakness leads to failure, and failure amounts to worthlessness. As survivors we've had our vulnerability exploited. Our trust and openness were taken and replaced with nearly unspeakable pain. The social mandates placed upon men and the emotional wounds that accompany sexual abuse combine to make the journey of fatherhood one that is both promising and perilous for male survivors. There are many questions that we ask ourselves with regard to fatherhood. What follows is a brief discussion about just a few of those questions.

Is this a trip that I really want to take? Parenting is a serious commitment that involves a lot of hard work. While many, including myself, find that the rewards more than justify the effort, it is important to note that parenting is not for everyone. Far too many become parents without taking the time to consider if, why, and when they really want to have children. Ideally everyone should know the answers to these questions before they enter into parenting, but if you and/or your partner are abuse survivors, they become even more important.

While social norms continue to evolve, the nuclear family with a mother, father, and one or more children, is still presented as the "normal" basic social unit of our culture. Most of us feel continuous gentle, and sometimes not-so-gentle pressure, to "settle down and have kids." Well-meaning friends and family often add to that pressure. Setting healthy boundaries and standing up for oneself can be tough for anyone, but as survivors many of us are taught our worth is based on our willingness and ability to please others. It can sometimes take years for a survivor to develop the power to "Just say no," but without this ability the decisions we make can never truly be voluntary.

As fulfilling as fatherhood has been for me, I commend those who make the conscious choice not to have kids and I feel it is important to include a discussion about this option. Fortunately I was recently able to speak with a good friend and fellow survivor about this. As my friend explained, when he considered having children, one thing that thing that he found attractive was that it would give him the opportunity to prove that he could be a better parent than his own parents had been to him. Ultimately, he came to the realization that, as he put it, "That's a really crappy reason to have a kid." While I appreciate his candor, the unfortunate reality is that far too many people have kids for even crappier reasons. My friend also explained that he and his wife like to go out, they like having money and they like being able to sleep in on weekends. For most, having children means having to give up at least some of perks that come with a pre-kid lifestyle. It's important to realistically assess both your and your partner's priorities and to respect each other's limits.

Am I destined to become an abuser myself? This is a question that unfairly haunts many survivor dads. The vampire myth covered elsewhere in this book is a horribly mistaken, yet widely held belief that men who were sexually abused as children are more likely to become abusers themselves. The idea is based on the misinterpretation and/or misuse of findings from research conducted with sex-offender populations. The body of research that can be appropriately applied to this question tells us that male survivors are no more likely to become abusers than are their non-abused peers. Unfortunately, just like nearly everyone else, we survivors have grown up hearing this myth repeated by friends, family, politicians, pastors, and the media, just to name a few. Is it any wonder that some of us are afraid to have children? Or, if we are not afraid to have them, then we are afraid of finding ourselves in certain situations with our kids? How many men refuse to change diapers? Sure, most of them are probably just being macho jerks or trying to get out of doing the dirty work, but sadly many of them are afraid to change diapers not because they are actually at risk of harming their kids, but because society has told them that they are. If you or your partner have these fears, even if the fears are completely unwarranted, they still need to be addressed. Ignoring them can severely impact your relationship.

Will others think I am abusing my kids? While some survivors are haunted by the vampire myth, many of us are very confident that we would never harm our children. Unfortunately, we are also well aware that a significant number of people will look upon us with suspicion. Of course most men, regardless of their survivor status, have had to deal with suspicion. Just ask any dad who has carried his kicking, screaming child out of a crowded shopping mall. For dads who are CSA survivors however, the problem takes on new dimensions. Male survivors are not "just being paranoid" or "overthinking things" when they experience concern over what others may think. The belief that male CSA survivors are likely to become perpetrators themselves is still common in society at large. Despite overwhelming evidence, the myth persists and harmful consequences for survivors continue. Scores of innocent men have been denied contact with their children due to baseless suspicions.

Do I have what it takes be a good father? Parenting is the most complicated job I know of that doesn't come with a manual. We are typically left to our own experiences and advice from the previous generation to figure out how to parent. Decades of social science research has only scratched the surface when it comes to our understanding of how to raise children. There are however, some things we know.

Beyond the basic needs of food, clothing, and shelter, our children need to feel safe and secure. Sometimes we survivors struggle with depression, anger, or anxiety. These unwanted emotions can often lead to behaviors that are unsafe, like substance abuse or physical violence, and still other behaviors that feel unsafe to those we love, such as excessive worry or anger. I have struggled with all of these unwanted emotions and behaviors over the years and while I have made a lot of progress, I still grapple with anger. I know that I can sometimes be a scary yeller and I don't want my son to grow up with memories of me like those that I have of my own father. I am fortunate to have a wife who is understanding and supportive.

As a partner, there is nothing you can do to make unwanted emotions go away, but you may help your survivor manage his behaviors related to those emotions. First, you need to keep yourself and your children safe. Do not tolerate physical violence or substance abuse. You also need to make your boundaries clear about which behaviors you will not tolerate. Beyond that, you can work with him to find healthy ways to cope with his unwanted feelings. This might include encouraging him to go to therapy, or to participate in a healthy activity that helps him sort through his emotions. There are support groups online that can help each of you; malesurvivor.org even has a forum just for partners.

Another thing that we know children need is healthy, affectionate touch. Some survivors have great difficulty with touch. In our experience affectionate touch has sometimes been anything but healthy and that causes some of us to avoid it all together. Children, of course, can't always understand that daddy doesn't like to be touched, and while it may be tempting to simply take on all of the snuggling duties yourself, it is nevertheless important for dads to be able to bond with their kids. Physical contact is an important piece of that. If the survivor you love is having trouble with this, he needs to know that he has your support. He may even need help learning how to be affectionate with a child, especially if he displays that stereotypical male fear of babies. A little gentle persistence can go a long way.

Finally, children need to build healthy self-esteem, and we parents need to provide an environment where they can do that. As survivors, many of us learned that our value as people was dependent on what we could do for others sexually. At an early age, our development of self-esteem was either stopped altogether or sent in an unhealthy direction. Even children who were not sexually abused were often raised with the idea that too much confidence is a bad thing. Confidence is a great thing; it is arrogance that we want to avoid. While it's fine to occasionally tell our kids, "You're so cute," or, "You're so smart," we should reserve the majority of praise for achievement involving effort and persistence. For example, "Wow, you worked really had at that, and you did it." Beyond learning the techniques, and overcoming misinformed views, survivors may also have to deal with issues that arise regarding unfairness. As parents most of us want to provide lives for are children that are as good, or better, than we had. Survivors are no different in this regard. For many of us however, there are moments when our children's lives remind us of the dysfunction in our own experiences. It seems counter-intuitive but sometimes seeing our kids happy can make us feel sad, as we mourn the loss of experiences that we missed. Your survivor needs to be able to experience these feelings before he can move past them. Often, all it takes is knowing that someone understands.

Can I still be strong for my children? Often, healing requires that we allow ourselves to fully experience emotions that we have previously suppressed. As men, coming to grips with the fact that we were once vulnerable children can be difficult under any circumstance. As fathers, we expect to be the protectors who make our kids feel safe. So, how do we process the emotional pain that was inflicted on the little boy so long ago while still projecting the strength and confidence that our kids need to see when they look to us for safety? I think the answer to this lies in the way we define strength vs. weakness. Pain is not weakness. Letting pain control your life is weakness. Allowing yourself to feel the pain, process it, and recover from it, is the true source of strength. If we take this to heart, our children will learn about true strength from our example.

Am I too protective? The internet and your local bookstore are filled with long-winded opinions from self-proclaimed experts about the dangers of being an overprotective parent. If you let them, these authors will convince you that "overprotectiveness" is the biggest problem in parenting today. Considering however, that roughly 20% of the population has been sexually abused as children and nearly two-thirds of us have suffered some form of significant adversity in childhood, I have to believe that the majority of us are not adequately protected as children. Beyond that, the term overprotective has no agreed upon definition within the research community. Very few quantitative studies have been done on the topic and I have yet to see scientific evidence of any damage done to children from protecting them too much. On the other hand, we have a mountain of research evidence linking childhood adversity (often an outgrowth of insufficient protection) to a long and growing list of negative outcomes.

That said, I will acknowledge that it might be possible to accidently limit a child's growth opportunities as a side effect of our efforts to protect them. Additionally, parents who have been abused as children frequently display hypervigilance as compared to their non-abused peers. If you are concerned that your survivor is too restrictive with your children, it's important to maintain open communication with him on this issue. Parents don't have to be in complete agreement on every detail of a kid's life, but they should be able to get close on the major stuff. My wife and I may disagree on the importance of our son wearing socks, but we trust each other enough that if either one of us feels uncomfortable with a situation, we can put the brakes on at any moment, and the other will respect that decision. That trust comes from the many honest and frank discussions we've had concerning our child's safety.

What are the upsides? Of course, every parent has a different experience. For some, myself included, raising our children is among the greatest joys we've ever known. Others feel it's the biggest mistake they've ever made. Most fall somewhere in-between the two extremes. In this regard, survivors are like anyone else, the happiness we gain from our parenting experience depends on the individual and the situation.

I refer to my own experience as parenting in reverse. The first time I became a father was the day I adopted two teenagers and a 9 year old. I immediately embarked on the odyssey that is being a father to three girls, with all of its challenges and rewards. Years later, my wife gave birth to our son. He is 7 years old now and I have had the privilege of seeing him grow from our little 8 pound bundle of joy into the much bigger bundle of joy we have today. And along with it were all of the diaper changes, spit-ups, and worries that are common to first-time parents.

As discussed above, survivors face unique challenges with regard to parenting but we also experience unique benefits. For most of my life, I carried immense amounts of guilt and shame, connected to my sexual abuse history. Beyond all reason, I blamed myself for what was done to me. "I was a smart kid," I reasoned. "How could I have let people take advantage of me like that?" My experience as a parent has helped me to erase all of that self-blame. Seeing the girls grow into and through their teens reminded me that even teenagers are still kids. They were not just small adults and neither was I at that age. And still today when I look into my son's face, I cannot possibly see him as anything other than the sweet, innocent, little kid that he is, and that I was too back then.

List of Contributors

Christopher Anderson, p. 131
MaleSurvivor.org

Melody Bacon, Ph.D., p. 241
The Chicago School of Professional Psychology

Nikeisha Brooks, M.A., p. 111
The Chicago School of Professional Psychology

Robert A. Carey, Psy.D., pp. 15, 349
County of San Bernardino, California
Dept. of Mental Health

Reginaldo Chase Espinoza, Psy.D. pp. 46, 54, 55, 58-60
The Chicago School of Professional Psychology

Crystal Flores, p. 117
The Chicago School of Professional Psychology

Ashley Fortier, M.A., p. 177
The Chicago School of Professional Psychology

Jennifer Harman, Ph. D., p. 167
Colorado State University

Loren M. Hill, Ph.D., p. 77
The Chicago School of Professional Psychology

Erin Langdon, M.A., pp. 149, 341
The Chicago School of Professional Psychology

Michael Levittan, Ph.D., p. 279
Private Practice

Matthew Love, Psy.D., p. 265
Fairfield University

Raymond Nourmand, Ph.D., p. 207
American Jewish University

Cris Scaglione, Ph.D., p. 197
The Chicago School of Professional Psychology

Richard S. Sinacola, Ph.D., p. 221
The Chicago School of Professional Psychology

Joshua D. Wyner, Ph.D., p. 329
The Chicago School of Professional Psychology

Adam F. Yerke, Psy. D., p. 177
The Chicago School of Professional Psychology

Consolidated List of References

Alaggia, R. (2005). Disclosing the trauma of child sexual abuse: A gender analysis. *Journal of Loss and Trauma, 10,* 453-470. doi: 10.1080/15320500193895

Alaggia, R., & Millington, G. (2008). Male child sexual abuse: A phenomenology of betrayal. *Clinical Social Work Journal, 36*(3), 265-275. doi:10.1007/s10615- 007-0144-y

Alaggia, R., & Mishna, F. (2014). Self psychology and male child sexual abuse: Healing relational betrayal. *Clinical Social Work Journal, 42*(1), 41-48.

Al Eissa, M., Almuneef, M. (2010). Child abuse and neglect in Saudi Arabia: Journey of recognition to implementation of national prevention strategies. *Child Abuse Neglect, 34* (2010), pp. 28-33

Al Jazeera. (2013, January 01). *Ndiyindoda: I am man.* Retrieved from Al Jazeera People and Power: http://www.aljazeera.com/programmes/peopleandp ower/2013/01/20131211736199557.html

Allen, K. (2006, July 25). *Bleak future for Congo's child soldiers.* Retrieved from BBC: http://news.bbc.co.uk/2/hi/africa/5213996.stm

Andersen, T. (2013). Against the wind: Male victimization and the ideal of manliness. *Journal of Social Work,* Vol. 13, (3), pp. 231-247.

Archer, J. (2000). Sex differences in aggression between heterosexual partners: A meta-analytic review. *Psychological Bulletin,* 126 (5), pp. 651-680.

Bailey, B. (2010). Partner violence during pregnancy: Prevalence, effects, screening, and management. *International Journal of Women's Health*, Vol. 2, pp. 183-197.

Banyard, P. &. (2011). *Ethical issues in psychology*. New York, New York: Routledge, Inc.

Bartholomew, K., Regan, K.V., White, M.A. & Oram, D. (2008). Patterns of abuse in male same-sex relationships. *Violence and Victims*. 23(5), 617-636.

Bartoloni, A. (2012, December 13). *Enduring scars: Child soldiers and mental health*. Retrieved from Irish forum for Global Health: http://globalhealth.ie/2012/12/13/enduring-scars-child-soldiers-and-mental-health/

Berkowitz, E. (1974). Some determinants of impulsive aggression. *Psychological Review, 81*: pp. 165-176.

Bettencourt, B. and Miller, N. (1996). Gender differences in aggression as a function of provocation: A meta-analysis. *Psychological Bulletin*, Vol. 119 (3), pp. 422-447.

Boscarino, J. A. (2004). Posttraumatic stress disorder and physical illness: results from clinical and epidemiologic studies. *Annals of the New York Academy of Sciences, 1032*(1), 141-153.

Braudy, L. (2003). From chivalry to terrorism: War and the changing nature of masculinity. New York: Alfred A. Knopf.

Brackenridge, C. (2001). Spoilsports: Understanding and preventing sexual exploitation in sport. London; New York; United Kingdom: Routledge.

Briere, J., & Scott, C. (2006). Principles of trauma therapy: A guide to symptoms, evaluation, and treatment. Thousand Oaks, CA: Sage Publications.

Brown, N. (2011). Holding tensions of victimization and perpetration: Partner abuse in trans communities. In J.L. Ristock's (Ed.), *Intimate partner violence in LGBTQ lives* (pp. 153-168). New York: Routledge Publishing.

Brown, T.N.T. & Herman, J.L. (2015). *Intimate partner violence and sexual abuse among LGBT people: A review of existing literature.* Retrieved from https://williamsinstitute.law.ucla.edu/research/viole nce-crime/intimate-partner-violence-and-sexual-abuse-among-lgbt-people/

Bullock, R. (2015, May 29). *A month with three initiates during the Xhosa circumcision ritual.* Retrieved from Africa Geographical Magazine: http://magazine.africageographic.com/weekly/issue-48/xhosa-circumcision-ritual-south-africa-its-hard-to-be-a-man/#sthash.4NvIcfjn.dpuf

Burri, A., Maercker, A., Krammer, S., & Simmen-Janevska, K. (2013). Childhood trauma and PTSD symptoms increase the risk of cognitive impairment in a sample of former indentured child laborers in old age. *PLoS ONE, 8*(2), e57826. http://doi.org/10.1371/journal.pone.0057826

Bütz, M. R. (1993), THE VAMPIRE AS A METAPHOR FOR WORKING WITH CHILDHOOD ABUSE. American Journal of Orthopsychiatry, 63: 426–431. doi:10.1037/h0079449

Capaldi, D.M., Kim, H.K., & Shortt, J.W. (2004). Women's involvement in aggression in young adult romantic relationships: A developmental systems model. In Putallaz, M. B. &Bierman, K. L. (Eds.), *Aggression, antisocial behavior, and violence among girls: A developmental perspective* (pp. 223–241). New York: Guilford.

Caplan, G. (1961). *An approach to community mental health.* New York: Grune & Stratton.

Centers for Disease Control and Prevention (2014). *The National Intimate Partner and Sexual Violence Survey,* https://www.cdc.gov/violenceprevention/nisvs/index.htm

Cho, H. (2012). Examining gender differences in the nature and context of intimate partner violence. *Journal of Interpersonal Violence,* Vol. 27, (13), pp. 2665-2684.

Collins, R. 2004. *Ritual interaction chains.* Princeton: Princeton University Press.

Cook, P. (2009). Abused Men: The hidden side of domestic violence. Westport, CT: Praeger.

De Lind van Wijngaarden, J. W. (2014). 'Part of the job': male-to-male sexual experiences and abuse of young men working as 'truck cleaners' along the highways of Pakistan. *Culture, Health & Sexuality,* 16 (5), 562-574.

Desai, S., Arias, I., Thompson, M. P., & Basile, K. C. (2002). Childhood victimization and subsequent adult revictimization assessed in a nationally representative sample of women and men. *Violence and Victims, 17*(6), 639-653.

Diamond, J. (1999). *Guns, germs, and steel: The fates of human societies.* New York: W.W. Norton & Company.

Dong, M., Anda, R. F., Felitti, V. J., Williamson, D. F., Dube, S. R., Brown, D. W., & Giles, W. H. (2005). Childhood residential mobility and multiple health risks during adolescence and adulthood: The hidden role of adverse childhood experiences. *Archives of Pediatrics & Adolescent Medicine, 159*(12), 1104-1110.

Douglas, E. and Hines, D. (2011). The helpseeking experiences of men who sustain intimate partner violence: An overlooked population and its implications for practice. *Journal of Family Violence,* Vol. 26, (6), pp. 473-485.

Downs, A. (2006). Velvet rage: Overcoming the pain of growing up gay in a straight man's world. USA: Da Capo Press.

Draucker, C. B., Martsolf, D. S., Ross, R., Cook, C. B., Stidham, A. W., & Mweemba, P. (2009). The essence of healing from sexual violence: A qualitative metasynthesis. *Research in Nursing & Health,* 32(4), 366-378.

Drexler, M. (2011). Life after death: Helping former child soldiers become whole again. Harvard School of Public Health.

Ehrensaft, M.K., Moffitt, T.E., & Caspi, A. (2004). Clinically abusive relationships in an unselected birth cohort: Men's and women's participation and developmental antecedents. *Journal of Abnormal Psychology,* 113, 258–271.

Federal Bureau of Investigation (FBI). (2010). *Hate crime statistics, 2009.* Retrieved from https://www2.fbi.gov/ucr/hc2009/index.html

Federal Bureau of Investigation (FBI). (2016). *Hate crime statistics, 2015.* Retrieved from https://ucr.fbi.gov/hate-crime/2015/home

Felitti, V.J. et al, Relationship of childhood abuse and household dysfunction to many of the leading causes of death in adults; *American Journal of Preventive Medicine,* Volume 14 , Issue 4 , 245–258

Felitti, V.J., Anda, R.F., Nordenberg, D., Williamson, D.F., Spitz, A.M., Edwards, V., Koss, M.P., et al. The relationship of adult health status to childhood abuse and household dysfunction. *American Journal of Preventive Medicine.* 1998; 14:245-258.

Finkelhor, D. (1984). *Child sexual abuse: New theory and research.* New York: Free Press.

Finkelhor, D., & Browne, A. (1988). Assessing the long-term impact of child abuse: A review and conceptualization. In L. Walker (Ed.), *Handbook on sexual Abuse of children* (pp. 55-71). New York: Springer.

Finkelhor, D, Gelles, R., Hotaling, G., and Straus, M. (1983). *The dark side of families: Current family violence research.* Los Angeles: Sage Publications.

FORGE. (2011). *Transgender domestic violence and sexual assault resource sheet.* Retrieved from http://www.avp.org/storage/documents/Training%20and%20TA%20Center/2011_FORGE_Trans_DV_SA_Resource_Sheet.pdf

Galovski, T., & Lyons, J. A. (2004). Psychological sequelae of combat violence: A review of the impact of PTSD on the veteran's family and possible interventions. *Aggression and Violent Behavior*, 477-501.

Gardiner, H. W. (2011). *Living across cultures: cross cultural human development* (5th ed.). Boston: Pearson Education.

George, M. J., & Yarwood, D. J. (2004). *Male Domestic Violence Victims Survey 2001: Main findings*. Retrieved from www.dewar4research.org/DOCS/mdv.pdf

Ghanim, D. (2012). Gender violence: Theoretical overview. In *Violence and Abuse in Society*. Oxford, England: Praeger.

Gobin, R. L. (2011). Partner preferences among survivors of betrayal trauma. *Journal of Trauma & Dissociation*, 13(2), 152-174.

Goodyear-Brown, P., Fath, A., & Myers, L. (2012). Child sexual abuse: The scope of the problem. In Goodyear-Brown, P. (Eds.), Handbook of child sexual abuse: Identification, assessment, and treatment (3-10). Hoboken, NJ: John Wiley & Sons.

Hamel, J. (2014). Gender inclusive treatment of intimate partner abuse: Evidence-based approaches. New York: Springer Publishing Company.

Hanson, R. (2013). Hardwiring happiness: The new brain science of contentment, calm, and confidence. New York: Harmony Books.

Hartill, M. (2005). Sport and the sexually abused male child. *Sport, Education and Society, 10*(3), 287-304, doi: 10.1080/13573320500254869

Henry, S. B., Smith, D. B., Archuleta, K. L., Sanders-Hahs, E., Nelson Goff, B. S., Reisbig, K. L., et al. (2011). Trauma and couples: Mechanisms in dyadic functioning. *Journal of Marital and Family Therapy*, 319-332.

Herdt, G. (1982). *Rituals of manhood: Male initiation in Papua New Guinea*. Berkeley, CA: University of California Press.

Herek, G.M. (2009). Hate crimes and stigma-related experiences among sexual minority adults in the United States. *Journal of Interpersonal Violence, 24*, 54–74. doi:10.1177/0886260508316477

Hines, D. and Malley-Morrision, K, (2005). *Family violence in the United States*. Los Angeles: Sage Publications.

Hoff, B. H. (2012, February 12). *CDC Study: More men than women victims of intimate partner physical violence, psychological aggression*. Retrieved from Stop Abusive and Violent Environments:
http://www.saveservices.org/2012/02/cdc-study-more-men-than-women-victims-of-partner-abuse/

Hyunkag, H. (2012). Examining gender differences in nature and context of intimate partner violence. *Journal of Interpersonal Violence,* Vol. 27, (13), pp. 2665-2684.

Ingalhalikar, M, et. al. (2014). Sex differences in the structural connectome of the human brain. Proceeding of the National Academy of Sciences of the United States of America, Vol. 111, (2), pp. 2665-2684.

James, R., & Gilliland, B. (2013). *Crisis intervention strategies* (7th Ed.). Pacific Grove, CA: Brooks/Cole.

James, S.E., Herman, J.L., Rankin, S., Keisling, M., Mottet, L., & Anafi, M. (2016). The Report of the 2015 U.S. Transgender Survey. Washington, DC: National Center for Transgender Equality.

Janosik, E. (1986). *Crisis counseling: A contemporary approach.* Monterey, CA: Jones and Bartlett.

Johnson, M. (2006). Control and conflict: gender symmetry and asymmetry in domestic violence. *Violence Against Women,* Vol. 12, (11), pp. 1003-1018.

Jones, W. (1968). The ABC method of crisis management. *Mental Hygiene,* 52, 87-89.

Kaiser Family Foundation. (2001). Inside-OUT: A report on the experiences of lesbians, gays and bisexuals in America and the public's views on issues and policies related to sexual orientation. Retrieved from https://kaiserfamilyfoundation.files.wordpress.com/2013/01/new-surveys-on-experiences-of-lesbians-gays-and-bisexuals-and-the-public-s-views-related-to-sexual-orientation-chart-pack.pdf

Kanel, K. (2015). *A guide to crisis intervention* (5th Ed.). Stamford, CT: Cengage Learning.

Karl, A., Schaefer, M., Malta, L. S., Dörfel, D., Rohleder, N., & Werner, A. (2006). A meta-analysis of structural brain abnormalities in PTSD. *Neuroscience & Biobehavioral Reviews, 30*(7), 1004-1031

Katz, J., Arias, I., & Beach, S. R. H. (2000). Psychological abuse, self-esteem, and women's dating relationship outcomes. *Psychology of Women Quarterly,* 24, 349-357.

Kelly, C.E. & Warshafsky, L. (1987, July). *Partner abuse in gay male and lesbian couples.* Paper presented at the Third National Conference for Family Violence Researchers, Durham, NH.

Kimmel, M. (2017). Angry white men: American masculinity at the end of an era. New York: Nation Books.

Koenen, K. C., Driver, K. L., Oscar-Berman, M., Wolfe, J., Folsom, S., Huang, M. T., & Schlesinger, L. (2001). Measures of prefrontal system dysfunction in posttraumatic stress disorder. *Brain & Cognition, 45,* 64-78.

Kohlberg, L. A. (1996). A cognitive-development analysis of children's sex role concepts and attitudes. In E. E. Maccoby (Eds.), Toward a feminist development of sex differences (p. 82-173). Stanford, CA: Stanford University Press.

Kret, M. and DeGelder, B. (2012). Reviews and perspectives: A review of sex differences in processing emotional signals. *Neuropsychologia Journal,* The Netherlands, Vol. 50, pp. 1211-1221.

Kuehnle, K. & Sullivan, A. (2003). Gay and lesbian victimization: Reporting factors in domestic violence and bias incidents. *Criminal Justice and Behavior,* 30(1), 85-96.

Landolt, M.A. & Dutton, D.G. (1997). Power and personality: An analysis of gay male intimate abuse. *Sex Roles, 37,* 335-359.

Leskin, L. P. & White, P. M. (2007). Attentional networks reveal executive function deficits in posttraumatic stress disorder. *Neuropsychology, 21*, 275-284.

Leslie, D. and Cavanough, M. (2005). *Current controversies on family violence.* Thousand Oaks, CA: Sage Publications.

Liberzon, I. & Sripada C. S. (2008). The functional neuroanatomy of PTSD: A critical review. *Progress in Brain Research, 167,* 151–169.

Lightdale, J. and Prentice, D. (1994). Rethinking sex differences in aggression: aggressive behavior in the absence of social roles. *Personality and Social Psychology Bulletin,* Vol. 20, (1), pp. 34-44.

Lisak, D. (1994). The psychological impact of sexual abuse: Content analysis of interviews with male survivors. *Journal of Traumatic Stress, 7*(4), 525-548. doi: 10.1002/jts.2490070403

Love, M. (2014). Sexual abuse of male children in sports: Factors impacting disclosure (Doctoral dissertation).

Lurito, J. (2001). Temporal lobe activation demonstrates sex-based differences during passive listening. *Neuroradiology,* Vol. 220, (1).

Marin, A. and Russo, N. (1999). Feminist perspectives on male violence against women in *What Causes Men's Violence Against Women.* Thousand Oaks, CA: Sage Publications, Inc.

Martin, C. L., Ruble, D. N., & Szkrybalo. J. (2002). Cognitive theories of early gender development. *Psychological Bulletin, 128*(6), 903-933. doi: 10.1037//0033-2909.128.6.903

McAlinden, A.-M. (2006). 'Setting 'Em Up': Personal, Familial and Institutional Grooming in the Sexual Abuse of Children. Social & Legal Studies, 15, 339-62.

McElroy, W. (1996). The unfair sex in Bender, D. et. al. *Family violence: Current controversies.* San Diego: Greenhaven Press, Inc.

McGuffey, C. (2013). Rape and Racial Appraisals: Culture, Intersectionality, and Black Women's Accounts of Sexual Assault. *Du Bois Review: Social Science Research on Race, 10*(1), 109-130. doi:10.1017/S1742058X12000355

Meis, L. A., Kehle, S. M., Barry, R. A., Erbes, C. R., & Polusny, M. A. (2010). Relationship adjustment, PTSD symptoms, and treatment utilization among coupled National Guard soldiers deployed to Iraq. *Journal of Family Psychology*, 560-567.

Mejia, X. E. (2005). Gender matters: Working with adult male survivors of trauma. *Journal of Counseling & Development, 83*(1), 29-40.

Merrill, G.S. & Wolfe, V.A. (2000). Battered gay men: An exploration of abuse, help seeking, and why they stay. *Journal of Homosexuality, 39*(2), 1-30. doi: 10.1300/J082v39n02_01

Meyer, I.H. (2003). Prejudice, social stress, and mental health in lesbian, gay and bisexual populations: Conceptual issues and research evidence. *Psychological Bulletin,* 129, 674-697. doi:10.1037/0033-2909.129.5.674

Mills, L. (2008). Violent partners: A breakthrough plan for ending the cycle of abuse. New York: Basic Books.

Mizen, R. and Morris, M. (2007). *On aggression and violence: An analytic perspective.* New York: Palgrave Macmillan.

Nalavany, B. A., & Abell, N. (2004). An initial validation of a measure of personal And social perceptions of the sexual abuse of males. *Research on Social Work in Practice, 14*(5), 368-378. doi: 10.1177/1049731504265836

National Alliance on Mental Illness (NAMI). (2016). *LGBTQ.* Retrieved from https://www.nami.org/Find-Support/LGBTQ

National Coalition of Anti-Violence Programs (NCAVP). (2016a). *Lesbian, gay, bisexual, transgender, queer, and HIV-affected hate violence in 2015.* Retrieved from http://www.avp.org/storage/documents/ncavp_hvr eport_2015_final.pdf

National Coalition of Anti-Violence Programs (NCAVP). (2016b). *Lesbian, gay, bisexual, transgender, queer, and HIV-affected intimate partner violence in 2015.* Retrieved from:http://avp.org/wp-content/uploads/2017/04/2015_ncavp_lgbtqipvreport .pdf

Neikta. (n .d.). *Sambia Tribe's initiation from boyz to men.* Retrieved from Orijin Culture: http://www.orijinculture.com/community/masculini sation-dehumanization-sambia-tribe-papua-guinea/

Nettle, D. (2007). Empathizing and systematizing: What are they and what do they contribute to our understanding of psychological sex differences. *British Journal of Psychology,* Vol. 98, (2), pp. 237-255.

New York State Office for the Prevention of Domestic Violence (2017). Website: http://opdv.ny.gov/faqs/index.html#maleandfemale perps.

Nugent, N., Christopher, N., Crow, J., Brown, L., Ostrowski, S., & Delahanty, D. (2010). The efficacy of early propranolol administration at reducing PTSD symptoms in pediatric injury patients: A pilot study. *Journal of Traumatic Stress, 23,* (2), 282-287.

O'Brien, C. K. (2015). Don't tell: Military culture and male rape. *Psychological Services,* 12 (4), 357–365.

O'Brien, M. J. (1991). Taking sibling incest seriously. In M. Q. Patton (Ed.), *Family sexual abuse: Frontline research and evaluation.* (pp. 75-92). Newbury Park, CA.: Sage Publications.

Pappas, G. K. (2001). "Males who have sex with males (MSM) and HIV/AIDS in India: The hidden epidemic. *AIDS and Public Policy Journal,* 16 (1), 4-17.

Pollack, W. (1998). *Real boys: Rescuing our sons from the myths of boyhood.* New York: Henry Holt and Company, LLC.

Ponce, A.N., Williams, M.K. & Allen, G.J. (2004). Experience of maltreatment as a child and acceptance of violence in adult intimate relationships: Mediating effects of distortions in cognitive schemas. *Violence & Victims.* 19(1), 97-108. doi: 10.1891/vivi.19.1.97.33235

Prado, J., Chadha, A., & Booth, J. R. (2011, November 1). The brain network for deductive reasoning: A quantitative meta-analysis of 28 neuroimaging studies. *Journal of*

Cognitive Neuroscience, 23(11), 3483-3497. http://dx.doi.org/10.1162/jocn_a_00063

Raison, C., & Miller, A. (2003). When enough is too much: The role of insufficient glucocorticoid signaling in the pathophysiology of stress related disorders. *American Journal of Psychiatry, 169,* 1554-1565.

Romano, E., & De Luca, R. V. (2001). Male sexual abuse: A review of effects, abuse characteristics, and links with later psychological functioning. *Aggression and Violent Behavior, 6*(1), 55-78.

Rothman, E. & Nnawulezi, N. (2016). Intimate partner violence, male. In A. Goldberg (Ed.), *The SAGE Encyclopedia of LGBTQ Studies* (pp. 467-468). Thousand Oaks, CA: SAGE Publications.

Sageman, S. (2003). The rape of boys and the impact of sexually predatory environments: Review and case reports. *Journal of the American Academy of Psychoanalysis, 31*(3), 563-580
. doi: 10.1521/jaap.31.3.563.22137

Salter, A.C. (1992). Transforming Trauma: A Guide to Understanding and Treating Adult Survivors of Child Sexual Abuse. Los Angeles: SAGE Publications, Inc; 1 edition

Schnarch, D. (2009). Passionate marriage: Keeping love and intimacy alive in committed relationships. New York: W.W. Norton & Co.

Schore A. N. (2000). Attachment and the regulation of the right brain. *Attachment and Human Development, 2*(1), 23-47.

Shapiro, F., & Forrest, M. (1997). *EMDR*. New York: Basic Books.

Sinacola, R. (2015, September). *The A-B-Cs of Trauma and Crisis Intervention*. Symposium presented at Pacific Oaks College, Pasadena, CA.

Sinacola, R., & Peters-Strickland, T. (2012). *Basic psychopharmacology for counselors and psychotherapists*. (2nd Ed.). Boston: Allyn and Bacon.

Sparato, J., Mullen, P. E., Burgess, P. M., Wells, D. L., & Moss, S. A. (2004). Impact of child sexual abuse on mental health. *The British Journal of Psychiatry*, 184(5), 416-421.

Stevens, J.E. (2012, October 3) ACES News, The-Adverse Childhood Experiences Study-The largest-most-important public health study you never heard of-began in an obesity clinic. Retrieved from https://acestoohigh.com/2012/10/03/the-adverse-childhood-experiences-study-the-largest-most-important-public-health-study-you-never-heard-of-began-in-an-obesity-clinic/

Stevens, M. J. (2007). Toward a global psychology: Theory, research, intervention, and pedagogy. Mahwah, NJ: Lawrence Erlbaum Associates, Inc.

Stojanovich, L., & Marisavljevich, D. (2008). Stress as a trigger of autoimmune disease. *Autoimmunity reviews*, 7(3), 209-213.

Stotzer, R.L. (2016a). Hate crimes. In A. Goldberg (Ed.), *The SAGE Encyclopedia of LGBTQ Studies* (pp. 467-468). Thousand Oaks, CA: SAGE Publications.

Stotzer, R.L. (2016b). Sexual minorities and violence. In A. Goldberg (Ed.), *The SAGE Encyclopedia of LGBTQ Studies* (pp. 1055-1058). Thousand Oaks, CA: SAGE Publications.

Stotzer, R.L. (2016c). Transgender people and violence. In A. Goldberg (Ed.), *The SAGE Encyclopedia of LGBTQ Studies* (pp. 1245-1246). Thousand Oaks, CA: SAGE Publications.

Straus, M. (1988). *Abuse and victimization across the lifespan.* Baltimore: Johns Hopkins University Press.

St-Yves, M. & Pellerin, B. (2002). Sexual victimization and sexual delinquency: Vampire or Pinocchio syndrome? Correctional Service Canada Forum, 14, 51-52.

Swarup, S. (2016, October 11). *Domestic violence against men.* Retrieved from merinews: http://www.merinews.com/article/domestic-violence-against-men/15920158.shtml

Taft, C. T., Stafford, J., Watkins, L. E., & Street, A. E. (2011). Posttraumatic stress disorder and intimate relationship problems: A meta-analysis. *Journal of Consulting and Clinical Psychology*, 22-33.

Tener, D., & Murphy, S. B. (2015). Adult disclosure of child sexual abuse: A literature review. *Trauma, Violence, & Abuse*, 16(4), 391-400.

Trenholm, J. O. (2013). Constructing soldiers from boys in Eastern Democratic Republic of Congo. *Men and Masculinities*, 16 (2), 203-227.

Valente, S. M. (2005). Sexual abuse of boys. *Journal of Child and Adolescent Psychiatric Nursing, 18*(1), 10-16. doi: 10.1111/j.1744-6171.2005.00005.x

Van Dam, C. (2001). *Identifying child molesters: Preventing child sexual abuse by recognizing the patterns of the offenders.* New York: Haworth Maltreatment and Trauma Press.

Van der Kolk, B. (1986). *Psychological trauma.* Washington, D.C.: American Psychiatric Association Press.

Van der Kolk, B. (2014). The body keeps score: Brain, mind, and body in the healing of trauma. New York: Penguin.

Van der Kolk, B., McFarlane, A. C., & Weisaeth, L. E. (1996). *Traumatic Stress: The effects of overwhelming experience on mind, body, and society.* New York: Guilford.

Veterans Affairs. (2013-2015). Military culture: Core competencies for healthcare professionals (Military organization and roles). Department of Veterans Affairs, Employee Education System and Department of Defense.

Walker, J., Archer, J., & Davies, M. (2005). Effects of rape on men: A descriptive analysis. *Archives of Sexual Behavior, 34*(1), 69-80. doi: 10.1007/s10508-1001-0

Weber, D. A., & Reynolds, C. R. (2004). Clinical perspectives on neurobiological effects of psychological trauma. *Neuropsychology Review, 14*(2), 115-129.

Weiner, Linda; Avery-Clark, Constance (2017). *Sensate Focus in Sex Therapy: The Illustrated Manual.* New York, NY: Routledge.

Wekerle, C. & Wolfe, D. A. (2003). Child maltreatment. In E. J. Mash, & R.A. Barkley (Eds.), *Child psychopathology* (2nd ed., pp. 632-683). New York: Guilford Press.

White, C. & Goldberg, J. (2006). Expanding our understanding of gendered violence: Violence against trans people and their loved ones. *Canadian Women's Studies, 25*(1-2), 124-127.

Whitfield CL. Adverse Childhood Experiences and Trauma. American Journal of Preventive Medicine. 1998; 14:361-363.

Whitman, C.N. & Nadal, K.L. (2016). Microaggressions. In A. Goldberg (Ed.), *The SAGE Encyclopedia of LGBTQ Studies* (pp. 768-770). Thousand Oaks, CA: SAGE Publications.

Xiong, Z. B., Tuicomepee, A., LaBlanc, L., & Rainey, J. (2006). Hmong immigrants' perceptions of family secrets and recipients of disclosure. *Families in Society: The Journal of Contemporary Social Services, 87*(2), 231-239.

Yerke, A.F. & DeFeo, J. (2016). Redefining intimate partner violence beyond the binary to include transgender people. *Journal of Family Violence, 31*(8), 975-979.

CPSIA information can be obtained
at www.ICGtesting.com
Printed in the USA
LVHW021520260619
622434LV00016B/626